VEGAN MEAL PREP:

TASTY RECIPES PLANT-BASED RECIPES INCLUDING DAY 1-30 OF MEAL PREP TO SAVING YOUR TIME

Dr Steven Green

TABLE OF CONTENTS

CONCLUSION...**226**

Introduction

Veganism is steadily gaining popularity, and for the right reasons. A vegan diet is devoid of any animal-based products, including eggs and dairy. Veganism is not just a diet but also a lifestyle choice. A vegan diet can help with weight loss, reduce the risk of certain diseases, and improve your energy levels. If you want to increase your chances of sticking to this diet, concentrating on the food you consume should be your priority.

Well-arranged vegan diets are viewed as suitable for all phases of life, including earliest stages and pregnancy by many medical schools and academies. Vegan diets will in general be higher in dietary fiber, magnesium, folic corrosive, nutrient C, nutrient E, iron, and phytochemicals; and lower in dietary vitality, immersed fat, cholesterol, long-chain omega-3 unsaturated fats, nutrient D, calcium, zinc, and nutrient B12.

The recipes in the book are for breakfast, lunch, dinner, and desserts using vegan ingredients. These recipes are not only easy to follow but will help you cook delicious and nutritious meals. You no longer have to compromise on taste for the sake of nourishment. Apart from this, you will also learn the basics of vegan meal prep, the benefits of meal prepping, vegan food lists that you should have handy, and tips for getting started today.

Once you start meal prepping, you can forget about takeout and fast food! You can start saving money, eating home-cooked meals, and improving your health. By using the different recipes given in this book, you can begin prepping meals like a pro. In today's world, it is quite easy to fall into the habit of eating fast food. Regardless of whether you are trying a plant-based diet or are weakened by choice, it can become a little challenging, since finding vegan options is not always easy. Are you ready to learn more about all this? If yes, then let us get started immediately. By the time you finish reading this book, you will feel encouraged knowing that you are prepared with all the tools you need to succeed!

Chapter 1: What is Vegan

A vegan diet is a strict form of the vegetarian diet that mandates eating only non-animal products. While vegetarians may afford themselves some wiggle room to eat something non-vegetarian once in a while, vegans typically don't use any products that contain any ingredients originating from or tested on animals.

A vegan will typically choose this diet because of health, ethical, or environmental reasons. If the person had health problems because of a diet rich in animal foodstuffs or opposes the unethical treatment of animals in the food industry or considers human exploitation of the environment over the top, then the vegan diet is the most appropriate solution.

A vegan diet is most often accompanied by but doesn't necessarily include the idea of toning down on consumerism. In other words, a vegan is an animal lover who rebels against the consumer culture and strikes his own path through the world. In other words, vegan is a hardcore vegetarian.

A vegan diet consists of a variety of colorful fruits and vegetables that almost beg to be showcased on all of the social media outlets and especially in your blog. The beautiful colors of common vegan dishes give off a vibrant, welcoming, and warm vibe that adds color to your day, diet, and even your favorite social media account. Well-known vegan bloggers have perfected taking photos of his/her overflowing bowls of vegan goodness.

Vegetarians do not consume meat or fish, but include other foods such as eggs and dairy products in their diet.

Vegan people have plenty to cook! I know when you start, there seems to be nothing to eat. Yet if you understand something, vegan food is fun, delicious, and nutritious. I don't feel like I'm missing anything.

Vegan diets consist only of vegetable-based foods, but vegans eat many of the same foods as non-vegans: pasta, rice, potatoes, salads, burgers, chips, tacos and even pizzas. Essentially, anything made from animal products can be vegan as well.

Whole grain products include spaghetti, bread, rice, quinoa, beans, meal and other whole grain products. However, whole grain diets make up a large part of your diet and provide a great deal of your protein, fats, complex carbohydrates, vitamins, and minerals.

Plant: A large part of your diet is made up of vegetables and omnivores. These are low in calories but high in fiber, organic, phytochemical, and satisfy many nutritional requirements.

The only plants you can eat every day are dark green leafy greens. You should also think about eating as many different colors of vegetables as possible on a regular basis.

It is recommended that you eat at least one salad a day and add more vegetables to your daily diet by adding them to smoothies, soups, stews, and everything else.

Fruit: Several portions of fruit a day are a fantastic way to better meet your nutritional needs, particularly to improve the intake of antioxidants for disease. Fruit is rich in calories, minerals, vitamins and phytochemicals.

You can eat fresh or frozen fruit to take advantage of the many health benefits of berries. The healthiest fruits you can enjoy are hops, lime, mango, banana, and strawberries, but every fruit is a good fruit!

How is it with the oils?

Refined fats from oils are not needed for optimal health, as the essential fats present in them are already available from the food sources of a healthy plant diet.

We will fulfill most of our essential fatty acid requirements by including avocados, olives, nuts and seeds in our diet while using other nutrients and fiber. The oil consumption should be kept to

Well, veganism is so much more than the sad stereotypes society has conjured up about them. These days, veganism is steadily gaining popularity and is present everywhere. Did you know that Tesla offers cruelty-free leather in their cars? Did you know that Burger King introduced a vegan meat patty, and KFC UK came up with an original vegan chicken burger? It certainly goes to show how popular veganism has become.

The vegan diet is a plant-based diet. It is quite similar to a vegetarian diet, except that it excludes eggs as well as dairy products along with other animal-derived ingredients. Any products derived from an animal, such as meat, milk, cheese, eggs, gelatin, and honey, are not included in a vegan diet. Anything that is made out of an animal or by an animal is not vegan. A lot of vegans don't eat foods that are also produced using animal products such as some wines as well as refined white sugar.

Veggie lover low-quality nourishment comprises packaged crisps, chips that are hot, with no milk chocolate and parts of candies, alleged'health bars' which are pressed with sugars and so on. Should you somehow be able to expend nourishments, as an instance, that all of the time and eat them rather than your proper suppers, you're damaging your body? Instead, you can choose to create your own vegetarian preparing strategies, by way of instance, without milk, low-sugar snacks, brownies, cakes, oat and nut cuts, so on., such as dates, dried organic goods, crisp all-natural goods, nuts, coconut oil, extra-virgin olive seeds, and oil. Experience your eating regimen in a judicious and continuous manner, and provide your body with the nutritional supplements that it requires.

In case you need to shed weight, the veggie lover diet is one of those good eating regimens which it is possible to adapt to perform as such. It's rash to choose a fad diet that's low in fat, saturated in leaves and supplements one feeling denied. It's possible to enjoy avocadoes, olive oil, seeds and nuts with this particular eating regimen - maybe not at all like most injury abstains from food now. You may likewise appreciate a range of gourmet, strong cooking so that you won't need to feel refused. By producing your own heavenly and strong veggie fan heating plans, you're guaranteeing you will stay happy and chemical with this eating regimen, instead of frustrated and grumpy.

So if the veggie lover diet offers you a great deal of sound nutritional supplements, provides your body sufficient sound fats and does not leave you feeling denied, alright say it is wise or indiscreet to drift down this pathway? I'd say it is savvy.

There are some long drag veggie fans who've been on the vegetarian diet as long as they can recall or for quite a very long moment. These people are always lean and thin and possess a solid, shiny composition along with also a get-up-and-go that most are desirous of. Not at all like injury eats, this eating routine is reasonable. Why? You won't feel denied since there are a lot of yummy choices to consume. You're able to enjoy a broad range of beautiful veggie-lover heating programs or dinner programs, which can be anything but hard to find in books, on the internet, or by vegetarian formula electronic publications. The health care benefits of the eating regimen can permit you to understand it is well-worth neglecting meat and meat products. Several have completed as such and therefore are moving to do so now. Could this be you?

Weight loss on the vegetarian diet is sheltered, educated and economical. So perhaps it's now a chance to drop the entirety of your injury diet musings and thoughts, and select rather a solid, veggie enthusiast way of life which can leave your life components happy, strong and well-supported.

The talk of whether the vegetarian diet is unfortunate or sound is not new. The majority of people may say that an individual that embraces veganism will probably be inadequate in fundamental supplements found obviously in animal products, to be particular, animal-based protein. These individuals treasure the certainty that milk can keep their bones strong and red meat will provide standard protein to your own muscles.

So determined by those two contrasts in evaluations, how could one determine whether the veggie lover diet is undesirable or solid? Everything boils down to, not things 'conclusion,' nevertheless instead, on powerful actualities, evidence, contextual investigations and fair accounts of real people.

Benefits of a Vegan Diet

In this section, let us look at the different benefits of a vegan diet.

Plenty of nutrients

If you are just getting started with a vegan diet, then it will undoubtedly be drastically different from the diet of an average American. You must ensure that your diet doesn't contain any animal-derived produce. A vegan diet consists of whole foods, vegetables, fruits, legumes, grains, nuts, and seeds. Almost all the foods contained in this diet are rich in different nutrients. Not only is the content of fiber quite high in them, but they are also rich in antioxidants, nutrients like potassium, magnesium, and vitamins A, C, and E. As long as your vegan diet isn't poorly planned, your body will get all the nourishment it requires.

Reduces the risk of certain types of cancers

According to the World Health Organization, the risk of about one-third of cancers can be reduced by following a vegan diet. The underlying factors that induce life-threatening cancers can be effectively managed through this diet. It is believed that a diet rich in fruits and legumes helps reduce the risk of colorectal cancer. Consuming plenty of soy-based products reduces the risk of breast cancer. Avoiding animal products altogether offers protection against cancer of prostate, colon, and breast.

Promotes weight loss

The consumption of plant-based foods helps speed up the process of weight loss when compared to other diets. Since the vegan diet primarily focuses on the consumption of whole foods, it helps with weight loss. All the fiber you consume tends to make you feel full for longer without being heavy on calories. Therefore, there is a natural reduction in your calorie intake. It not only helps with weight loss but also improves your overall energy levels. A vegan diet isn't usually calorie-restrictive and encourages the consumption of whole foods that will leave you feeling full. Once the calorie intake reduces, it is easy to maintain a calorie deficit. A calorie deficit is quintessential for weight loss. Also, it is a great way to tackle cravings for unhealthy foods.

Stabilizing blood sugar

A vegan diet helps reduce the risk of type II diabetes while improving the health of your kidneys. The insulin secreted by the pancreas required to balance blood sugar levels reduces whenever the blood sugar levels reduce. It, in turn, reduces the risk of diabetes. By reducing the risk of diabetes, and managing blood sugar levels, the overall function of kidneys improves.

Managing inflammation

A vegan diet can help reduce as well as manage the uncomfortable pain caused by arthritis. Inflammation is the leading cause of arthritis. A diet that's rich in processed sugars and unhealthy carbs increases the chances of inflammation. Since a vegan diet doesn't concentrate on these two types of foods, inflammation can be easily managed. Once inflammation is managed, it becomes easier to regulate pain as well.

Risk of heart diseases decreases

Consuming a diet that's rich in vegetables, legumes, fruits, and other dietary fibers help reduce the risk of several heart diseases. It also helps regulate high blood sugar. It, in turn, helps reduce the risk of several cardiovascular disorders, while improving the overall functioning of the heart. A vegan diet helps reduce the level of LDL cholesterol within the body. HDL and LDL are two cholesterol molecules present within your body. HDL stands for high-density lipoprotein, and LDL stands for low-density lipoprotein. A lipoprotein helps carry cholesterol molecules in the body. The composition of the cholesterol molecules is pretty much the same, but the functions they perform are quite different. HDL is responsible for transporting cholesterol molecules away from the body. So, a low level of LDL and a high level of HDL is directly associated with a reduction in the risk of cardiovascular disorders.

By shifting to a vegan diet, you can effectively improve your overall health and wellbeing. Not just this, you can also attain your weight loss and fitness objectives too!

How the vegan diet works

The vegan diet is a strict vegetarian diet. Vegan not only prohibits meat and fish, but also dairy products such as milk, eggs and gelatin, as well as animal foods such as honey.

Like all other types of eating, the same applies to vegan diets. The best combination of nutrients is a diverse selection of different foods.

Significant sources of non-vegan iron, calcium, iodine, vitamin D and B12 are animal foods such as meat, fish and dairy products. The following foods are therefore important for a healthy vegan diet: good sources of iron are green vegetables such as chard and spinach, legumes such as lentils and beans, and grain products such as oatmeal.

Among green vegetables and herbs such as broccoli, fennel, basil, and petroleum, essential calcium is extracted. Calcium is also found in nuts and seeds such as hazelnuts and sesame.

Iodine mainly provides sea-living food. With vegan diets, algae or iodized table salt works well.

In addition to animal products, in fermented products such as sauerkraut and beer, vitamin B12 is also found in trace components. For example, in mushrooms, vitamin D is found, but is also produced by the body itself.

Only a few people understand what a vegan diet is or what it can mean for their health. Instead of a diet rich in fruits and vegetables, the typical American diet is rich in meat, fat and dairy. This way of eating has worsened with each generation. As this trend grows, so do the waistlines of many people. Instead, a vegan diet is a healthy alternative. Whether you eat vegan food for a short time or continue a lifetime, veganism can be a valuable lifestyle change.

The vegan diet is famous for its health benefits and especially for weight loss. Many people have made a vegan diet to lose weight and have succeeded.

Lose weight, enjoy more energy, and feel good by making a difference in vegetarianism. But before starting a vegan diet, you may be looking for a healthy and healthy diet to lose weight, and there are some things you should understand.

At first glance, it seems very difficult to follow a vegan diet. Animal products are everywhere, from gelatin to chocolate. Make many foods that you would not expect from animal products. In some parts of the world, choosing a vegan diet is very difficult.

If you plan the vegan diet sensibly and politely, you can be sure that it is safe and healthy. You need to ensure that you are eating a variety of different foods every day to ensure that you are receiving optimal nutrition - but hey, you need to do this on any diet. If you regularly eat vegan junk food, obviously your health is suffering.

So based on these two differences in opinions, how can one determine whether the vegan diet is healthy or unhealthy? It all comes down to, not matters of 'opinion,' but rather, on solid facts, evidence, case-studies, and truthful stories of real people.

Vegan diets often provide the body with much healthier vitamins and minerals as fresh fruits and vegetables substitute high-energy foods such as meat and sausages.

Vegan diet is an issue because food choices are one-sided and the opportunity for under-nutrition is too little awareness. Nutrients such as vitamin B12 are urgently required, especially during pregnancy and lactation and during childhood. Third, dietary supplements can be of help to your vegan diet.

Different types of vegan diet

- Ovo lacto vegetarians do not eat fish or meat. For example, they also do without gelatin, but eat products from live animals such as milk and honey.

- Lacto-vegetarians avoid meat, fish and eggs.

- Ovo vegetarians do without meat and fish as well as milk and milk products.

- Pescetarians do not eat meat, but fish.

- Frutarians want plants to be harmed as little as possible. They mainly eat fruit and nuts.

- Flexitarians are occasional vegetarians who value healthy food but do not continuously avoid meat or fish. (AP)

Chapter 2: What is Meal Prep

The preparation of meals is considered the universal solution with which we all can eat healthy, even under time pressure.

A meal plan is a practical organizational aid in everyday life: you think about what you cook, keep these thoughts in writing, write the best immediately a matching shopping list - and then you have the mind free and many carefree morning hours.

Healthy nutrition works easier with organization, because healthy food is not just a matter of ingredients but also of the organization. If I think about what I'm cooking in good time, there will be fewer emergency solutions - fast food.

It is addictive to cook. It is about keeping the seasonal fruits and vegetables and filling the storage cupboards in the heat. And then in the winter to eat cinnamon prunes of semolina pudding or fermented vegetables from the garden...

Advantages of having a meal plan

Saves Time

Preparing the meal plan requires a little time, but the time you can save is much longer. How many times have you asked yourself, what will I cook this day? What will I prepare for dinner? With a plan ready, this dilemma no longer exists. Each time you start working immediately. In addition, by having the list, you significantly shorten the time needed to make purchases.

Saves money

Meal planning helps you avoid impulse purchases. With a good shopping list you need only one or two visits to the store each week. In addition, it allows you to make better use of discounts, because you know the quantity and type of products you will need in the coming days.

Takes care of your health

Planning all meals of the day will help you eat healthier. You will avoid going for fast foods, which most contain preservatives and other harmful ingredients for us. Homemade food of fresh ingredients is the most beneficial solution.

Make a healthier choice

Whenever you eat out, you are likely to exceed your daily calorie and sodium intake! Just dropping in at a grocery store to have dinner at the last minute can result in insufficient options. When shopping on an empty stomach, you are more likely to put junk food in your cart.

Improve Nutrition

By planning ahead, you can have a nutritionally balanced diet throughout the week. For example, you can verify that each dinner has the necessary vegetables, protein, and grains. By planning a meal, you can ultimately control your personal nutritional needs. Whether you need to stick to a low sodium diet or just want to eat whole grains and vegetables, you can plan!

Eat high quality food

Homemade meals are often nutritious and are filled with fewer calories, salt, and fat than grocery store takeout's and simple ready-made options. A stand out advantage is you get to choose what you want as recipes will help you select important foods, such as buying local meat and organic produce.

Reduce stress

By making a meal plan, you can no longer throw away the forgotten ingredients in the refrigerator. You can create a meal plan that can use everything in the cupboard.

You can also start anew by creating a grocery list based on your meal plan. This allows you to go to the grocery store with a purpose rather than a whim. Also, do not serve dozens of unhealthy foods at random, but rarely eat them.

How to start planning meals?

1. Make a list of 15-20 of your favorite foods To make this list, sit down with your whole family and ask everyone about their favorite foods. Once this is done, look at the list and select those foods that are easy and quick to prepare and do not need too many ingredients.

The best if they are healthy meals.

2. Gather the recipes of the meals you are going to prepare Organize your list. You can divide the meals into groups, for example: soups, meat dishes, vegetarian dishes and so on, so that it is easy to handle them.

Find the recipes you need and write them down or print them on sheets of paper. Also, you may consider buying a special notebook for recipes. The most important thing is to have easy access to them, because you will need them often.

3. Plan all-day meals

Don't just create a list of lunches. It is advisable to eat 3-5 times a day, so think about planning all breakfasts, lunches and dinners.

This will avoid eating out, it will help you plan and use your cooking time better. You will also have the opportunity to make better use of food leftovers (it is important if you want to maximize the savings effect).

4. Write your menu on paper You have many ways to do it. Personally I use the template "weekly meal plan". Another way is to use a notebook. On the left side of the page you write a list of your meals, and on the right write all the necessary ingredients to prepare this meal (at one time you will have a meal plan and the shopping list).

5. Check what you have in your pantry Before putting your menu into action, it is a good idea to check your pantry, refrigerator and freezer first.

6. Adjust the menu according to your family's eventualities When you are planning meals, consider your daily activities and those of your family. Did your

children eat lunch at school? That day plan a more modest lunch at home. Do you come back late from work? Think of a dinner that takes little time to prepare. Has the family been invited to a Sunday dinner? You don't have to prepare dinner that day.

7. Use the seasonal products Depending on the season, the availability of individual fruits and vegetables can change dramatically. Therefore, their prices also change. The best prices will be found during the harvest, which becomes savings.

8. Prepare more meals at once Do you think about eating the same dish more than once in the week? Try to prepare a larger amount of this meal, for today and the next few days. If you do, put the food separately in containers and place them in the refrigerator or freezer, You can also bottle the food in jars.

9. Plan your food cleaning day If at the end of the week you collect all the leftovers from your refrigerator, you can plan a night, when together with your family you will have dinner only leftovers.

10. Review your daily plan

Your meal plan must be flexible. If necessary, don't be afraid to make modifications and use the opportunities.

Tips for creating a meal plan

A meal plan tells you which dishes or recipes you are considering for each meal. Use the calendar to plan each meal in the week or month. Look at the Food Hero recipes because each recipe has a "Make It a Meal" section where you can get ideas!

- ***It includes his family***. Collect recipes for healthy meals that your family enjoys and prepare them regularly. Invite your family to contribute ideas or plan meals with topics like " Friday night pizza ."

- ***Take it easy.*** Do not try to do too much. Includes recipes for fast foods , such as grilled sandwiches with vegetable salad, for those days when you know you won't have much time to cook.

- **_Use leftovers._** Think about how you can use a food more than once. Remains of cooked chicken on Monday could go on Tuesday's salad. Soups, stews, and peppers often taste even better the next day. They also freeze well.

- **_Seek inspiration:_** Talk to other people and look at magazines, cookbooks, newspapers and websites to get new ideas about meals and new recipes. Save the recipes and menus that your family enjoys, and redeem your favorites with other family members, friends, and neighbors.

- **_Cooking without meat_**: Try to include some recipes that include vegetable proteins, such as beans, lentils or tofu, which are usually cheaper than meat

- **_Keep a balance:_** Try to cover all food groups at daily meals and snacks: grains, vegetables, fruits, dairy, and protein. Try to plan a meal with all the food groups. When you're done, try the Super Tracker to see how healthy it is.

- ***Save preparation time.*** It includes recipes that have ingredients in common - for example, onions and brown rice. Then chop several onions and cook enough rice for two meals.

Steps Involved in Meal Prep

Now that you know what meal prepping is, it is time to get started. There are three important steps involved in meal prep, and they are as follows.

Identifying your needs

Before you start prepping, you need to understand your needs and requirements. Meal prepping makes it easier to cook meals. So, what are the different things you will need to do to ensure you feel more in control of the food you eat? Think about all the pain points associated with mealtime. Do you need to cook a healthy lunch you can carry to work? Do you wish to stock up on vegan snacks? Do you want to stop spending a lot of money on breakfast?

Selecting the right foods

Selecting the foods, you want to prep ahead to meet your needs is the second step. It certainly sounds quite easy, doesn't it? You might want to eat healthier breakfast, a light lunch, or perhaps a quick dinner. However, where do you start? Well, this is exactly where this book comes in. It presents plenty of meal prep ideas as well as recipes you can start using.

Creating a plan

Once you are aware of all that you wish to cook ahead, this is what you will need to do next. Start making a list of all the tasks you want to accomplish within the meal prepping time you have set aside. Make a list of items you will need to cook and think of ways in which you can multitask. Perhaps you can cook something on the stovetop while another item is baking in the oven.

When all the prep is done, you must portion and store it! Store them in the right containers, label them if you want, and keep it in the fridge or the freezer. By following these steps, meal prepping will become incredibly simple. It will no longer seem overwhelming even if you never tried it before. All the effort that you put in will certainly be worth it.

Meal Prep Tips

Whether you are just getting started with a vegan diet or are in it for the long haul, reducing the cooking time makes all the difference. Purchasing a ready-made meal from the veggie section of a supermarket certainly doesn't hurt once in a while, but it is always better to eat fresh and healthy meals. It is where meal prep steps in. Here are some simple tips you can start using to make vegan meal prep easy.

Frozen Foods

Frozen foods are as good as fresh produce. At times, there might not be sufficient time to wash, peel, or prep any fresh produce. So, try opting for frozen foods in such a case. They contain all the nutrients that fresh produce does. When it comes to cooking, you merely need to cook the frozen ingredients, and a meal will be ready within no time.

A Little Planning

Always plan before you start shopping for the required groceries. If you head to the grocery store without a list of ingredients you need, you will not only end up wasting your money but might also forget to pick the ingredients you want to cook with. So, spend some time and make a plan for all the meals you want to have in a week. Use the different recipes given in this book for a better idea.

Preparing Whole Grains

Cooking grains does take some time, and after a long day, you might not want to spend hours cooking in the kitchen. So, over the weekend, you can cook whole grains such as barley, quinoa, brown rice, or even couscous and store it for later. Once you have cooked the whole grains, lentils, and legumes, you merely need to store it in the fridge. You can easily reheat them along with some veggies!

Batch Cooking

One of the main components of meal prepping is batch cooking. If you're not used to cooking big portions, then now is the time to start. For instance, you can make a big pot of chili or any soup you like and repurpose the leftovers on other days. Certain items like broths, soups, and curries are best suited for batch cooking.

Individual Portions

Instead of baking a loaf of zucchini bread or a large casserole, start cooking recipes in individual portions. For instance, instead of a loaf tray, you can use a muffin pan! Batching cooking helps save time, but to make things easier, store the cooked food in individual serving sizes. Instead of storing curry in a huge container, store individual servings in storage bags. It certainly helps make meal prep easier.

Use a Slow Cooker

If you have a slow cooker or an instant pot, it is time to start using them frequently. If you don't, maybe you should consider investing in one. There are countless recipes you can cook using a slow cooker, and it is not just for making stews. All that you need to do is toss in the ingredients in the cooker, turn it on, and wait for it to work its magic. A slow cooker comes in handy, especially when you want to cook large portions.

Nut Butter

Start making different nut butter at home. It is quite easy to make almonds, sunflower seeds, cashews, or even peanut butter at home. You merely need to blend the nuts or seeds along with some oil, sugar, and salt. If you don't want to make it at home, you can always purchase them. Nut butter goes well with fruit, crackers, bread, carrots, and celery. Whenever hunger strikes, these nut butters will come in handy.

Using Leftovers

If you don't think you'll have time to prepare more than one meal at a time, cook multiple servings of it and then refashion it into different meals. Alternatively, you can also take elements from one meal and reuse them the next day. Leftovers from a taco can be repurposed into a pie, or leftover quinoa can be added to a salad. Leftovers certainly come in handy while prepping meals.

Fill Up on Snacks

You can have snacks for dinner as well. Whenever you are in a rush, a simple salad is a great snack. All that you need to do is merely some fruits and vegetables and top it with a simple salad dressing. Or you can even make some dips like tahini, hummus, baba ganoush, or salsa and serve it with crudités.

Right Containers

If you want to cook in batches or cook multiple portions of the same item, then you need to have the proper containers to store them. Keep in mind your favorite dishes while doing meal prep. Always opt for reusable containers instead of disposable ones. It certainly helps save time and money, not to mention that they are environment-friendly as well.

Use Canned Foods

Start using canned foods as well. A lot of people tend to look down on canned foods, but using them certainly saves time. Instead of cooking beans from scratch, opt for canned beans. The same applies to tomatoes as well. You merely need to rinse and heat the canned ingredients!

Safety and Storage Steps

With meal prepping, you need to ensure that you store the food safely. For instance, the food you store in the refrigerator must be consumed within 2 to 3 days. If you think you will need a while longer, then always store in the freezer. The risk of food poisoning is considerably lower when using plant foods rather than animal-based ones. It is primarily because bacteria thrive on protein-rich foods when compared to sugars and starches. However, rice and quinoa are certain exceptions to this rule. Therefore, take a little extra care while storing and reheating these foods. Before you begin, check whether the food is safe to eat or not.

By simply smiling and looking at it, you'll get the idea of it.

Before you store the food in the fridge, ensure that it is at room temperature. Never leave hot food in the refrigerator. If you place warm food in the refrigerator, it increases the overall temperature present within and increases the risk of other food getting spoiled as well. If you are using any frozen foods, ensure that it is at room temperature before you consume it. So, defrosting is essential.

Chapter 3: Benefits of Vegan Meal Prep

Who wouldn't want to lead a healthier life and feel more energized and fit? Well, everyone would want this. However, life can get a little hectic. Setting healthy goals is quite easy, but following through and staying on track becomes a little tricky. While you are busy navigating the hectic schedule of your daily life, the thought of cooking all your meals on your own is certainly not appealing. Not to mention the difficulty in thwarting off the temptations of eating out or ordering a meal. If you are tired of eating unhealthy junk food and want to eat healthier while saving some money, then meal prepping is the answer you have been looking for. In this section, let us look at some of the benefits of meal prep.

Grocery Shopping

Once you are aware of all the different meals you will be eating in a week, it becomes easier to shop for groceries. You no longer have to wander around aimlessly looking for inspiration or ideas to decide what to eat. Use the food list discussed in this book to prepare a grocery-shopping list. You can start dividing the list into different categories like vegetables, fruits, nuts and seeds, frozen foods, fats, and dairy alternatives. It also helps ensure that you don't give in to the temptation of buying unnecessary, processed foods.

Light on the Pocket

It is not expensive to start eating healthy. In fact, you might end up saving quite a lot of money. Once you start cooking all your meals at home. The only expenses you will incur are the ones towards shopping for groceries. Once you have everything you need to cook with, cooking becomes a breeze. Also, by planning all the meals, you will know what to buy and avoid making any unnecessary trips to the grocery store. When you know there is food waiting for you, it becomes easier to stop ordering meals.

Portion Control

An important skill you will learn once you start meal prepping is portion control. With meal prep, you will be dividing the food you cook into individual portions. By storing them in different containers, the urge to reach out for more or overindulge will be reduced. If weight loss is one of your priorities, then you need to consume sufficient nutrients. Portion control will help with this. You can certainly treat yourself occasionally, but learning to become mindful of the portions you eat is quintessential.

Weight Loss

When you know what you will be eating and how much you have to eat, you will automatically become mindful of the foods you consume. Weekly meal prep makes it easier to regulate the calories you consume daily. Since most of your meals will be home-cooked, you have complete control over the quality of ingredients you use. So, it is not just the quantity, but also the quality of the food you consume that improves as well. You don't necessarily have to count calories, but by substituting unhealthy ingredients with healthier alternatives, you can improve your overall health as well.

Less Wastage

Were there instances when you probably had to throw away produce because it expired or went bad before you had a chance to eat it? Wasting food is never a good feeling. It's not just a waste of money, but it is not environmentally sustainable. When you start meal prepping, you can make the most of all the ingredients you purchase. If you plan your meals correctly, you will be able to repurpose leftovers as well.

Saves Time and Effort

It does take a little time to plan and prepare meals in advance, but it is certainly worth the while. If you can dedicate a couple of hours over the weekend or whenever you are free to do the basic meal prep, cooking during the weekdays certainly becomes easier. Think about all the time you might usually end up worrying about what you will need to eat for your next meal. Once all your meals are prepared and planned, all that you need to do is reheat them and enjoy delicious and nutritious food.

Reduces Stress

Stress hurts your overall health. It not only weakens your immune system but also affects your sleeping pattern and digestive processes. Imagine how stressful it is when you come home after a hectic day and have to start thinking about what you need to eat for dinner. All this stress will be a thing of the past with meal prep. You can relax knowing that there is food ready when you go home.

Investment in Health

One of the great things about meal prep is that you can choose what you will be eating, and do this ahead of time. All those who follow meal prepping tend to eat cleaner than those who don't. You don't have to waste time finding something vegan to eat and risk eating unhealthy options because your meal is not ready. Eating healthy and well-balanced meals will undoubtedly improve your overall health. Proper nutrition is key to leading a healthy life.

Plenty of Variety

By putting a little thought into the kind of meals you will be eating, it becomes easier to select from different categories of foods like proteins, vegetables, fruits, and so on. When you plan, you can easily include the different food groups your body requires to all your meals. Apart from this, meal prep also encourages you to get creative with the recipes you use.

Better Willpower

Once you get into the groove of healthy eating, cravings for unhealthy foods and processed sugars will reduce. As your body gets used to the diet and the concept of healthy eating, it becomes easier to stay away from foods you know you must avoid.

Keep in mind that there is no right or wrong way to go about meal prepping. You have plenty of freedom to decide what you want to do. The best way to meal prep is via trial and error. After a week or two, you will quickly realize what works best for you.

Healthy plant power without cholesterol

Foods with animal ingredients are often unhealthy. This is partly due to the mostly unhealthy preparation, but also due to the composition of animal products. Substances that are problematic to health, such as cholesterol, saturated fatty acids or purines, are increasingly found in animal products, while they are present in much smaller quantities or not at all in plants. In addition, many health-promoting ingredients, such as fiber and phytochemicals, are only ingested through plants.

Improved sleep

Sleep is essential. Good sleep is essential, especially in a busy everyday life. Your body and mind need to regenerate at night and recharge your batteries. Since you cannot need long sleep or not sleep through! At this point, meal prep vegan comes in handy, because: Many types of vegetables and nuts contain vitamin B6, tryptophan and magnesium, which have a positive effect on sleep.

Chapter 4: List of Nutrient Rich Vegan Food

Regardless of whether you have been a vegan for a while or are trying out the vegan diet, you will undoubtedly come across several people who will seem skeptical of all that you are doing. A lot of people also believe that a vegan diet is extremely restrictive and limited. Does all this sound a little familiar? Well, if you were worried about these things, you can put your fears to rest. If you take a closer look, following a plant-based diet is quite simple. There are hundreds of options available. A vegan diet includes fruits, vegetables, nuts, seeds, grains, legumes, and a variety of other ingredients. It is quite easy to cook delicious meals without using any animal-based products.

Veganism is steadily gaining popularity, and these days there are various vegan-friendly products available in the market. From vegan meats to vegan dairy products, you don't have to worry about giving up on the foods you enjoy. By merely replacing certain ingredients, you can start enjoying all sorts of foods. Also, the different recipes given in this book will undoubtedly come in handy!

Being a vegan has become quite easy and convenient these days. To give you an overview of the limitless possibilities available, here is a vegan food list you can use.

Vegetables

You are free to consume as many vegetables as you want. Most of the vegetables are low in calories and rich in dietary fiber, phytonutrients, antioxidants, minerals, and vitamins that your body needs. You can use fresh as well as frozen vegetables.

The vegetables you can include are avocados, artichokes, asparagus, bell peppers, beetroot, broccoli, cabbage, brussels sprouts, cauliflower, carrots, cherry tomatoes, celery, collard greens, eggplant, cucumber, corn, peas, green beans, olives, jalapenos, mushrooms, okra, radishes, pumpkins, potatoes, shallots, squash, fennel, onions, chilies, peppers, potatoes, sweet potatoes, rhubarb, sprouts, zucchini, turnips, yams, and parsnips. The greens you can include are kale, spinach, Swiss chard, bok choy, arugula, lettuce, mixed salad leaves, watercress, endives, and so on.

You can pretty much include any vegetables that you want, including any which haven't been mentioned in this list.

Fruits

Fruits are rich in antioxidants, minerals, enzymes, vitamins, and other phytonutrients. They pretty much include all the good stuff that your body needs. The simple sugars present in fruits also give your body a quick boost of energy. You can use fresh, frozen, or even dried fruits.

The different fruits you can include are mango, pineapple, guava, pomegranate, kiwi, dragon fruit, apples, pears, plums, grapes, oranges, nectarines, bananas, watermelon, persimmon, mangosteen, lime, lemon, figs, apricots, prunes, peaches, honeydew melon, cantaloupe, jackfruit, lychees, cucumber, coconut, clementine, currants, durian, and grapefruit.

Berries are low in calories and rich in antioxidants and vitamins. There are various berries to choose from, like blackberries, blueberries, strawberries, goji berries, cranberries, mulberries, raspberries, and so on.

Starchy Items

Starches are rich in complex carbs that supply your body with energy while filling up your tummy. Apart from this, they contain plenty of proteins, fibers, minerals, and amino acids. Whenever you are purchasing starches, stick to whole grains instead of the processed ones.

The different whole grains, you can include are rye, buckwheat, millet, quinoa, oats, wheat, wild rice, corn, barley, amaranth, whole wheat, bulgur, farro, kamut, millet, and einkorn. Apart from whole grains, you can also consume a variety of legumes. The different legumes you can start adding to your diet are pinto beans, black-eyed peas, black beans, chickpeas, fava beans, lentils, mung beans, navy beans, white beans, red beans, split peas, snow peas, sugar snap peas, soybeans, alfalfa sprouts, cannellini beans, azuki beans, lima beans, kidney beans, and green beans.

Herbs and Spices

Herbs and spices not only help elevate the flavors of the food you consume but are also good for your health. Most of the herbs and spices tend to have anti-inflammatory properties. Regardless of whether you are using fresh or dried herbs, they are a great way to improve your overall health. While following a vegan diet, you can include all herbs and spices. For instance, you can add cilantro, bay leaf, star anise, basil, chamomile, celery, chili powder, chives, coriander, dill, garlic, ginger, lemongrass, nutmeg, nutritional yeast, onion powder, oregano, peppermint, pepper, parsley, mint, time, turmeric, saffron, rosemary, red pepper flakes, poppy seeds, and paprika.

Healthy Fats

All fats are not created equal. There are some unhealthy fats and some extremely healthy ones. Saturated fats and trans fats are undesirable and are the reasons why fats tend to get a bad rap. However, the fats present in whole plant foods are extremely good for the overall functioning of your body. They enable the proper development as well as the functioning of the nervous system, improve the absorption of nutrients, and promote the heart's health. Including a variety of healthy, plant-based fats provides Linoleic acid and alpha-linolenic acids. Consuming sufficient healthy fats ensures that there exists a balance between omega-3 fatty acids and omega-6 fatty acids in your body. However, you need to be mindful of the fat consumption.

The different sources of healthy fats include nuts, seeds, and butter made from various nuts and seeds. You can start adding chia seeds, hemp seeds, flax seeds, sesame seeds, sunflower seeds, pumpkin seeds, cashews, pistachios, almonds, Brazil nuts, chestnuts, macadamia nuts, hazelnuts, walnuts, and pine nuts to your daily diet. Other sources of healthy fats include avocados, olives, and oils made from these ingredients.

Condiments and Miscellaneous Items

The different condiments you can include are salsa, mustard, hummus, harissa, coconut milk, baked beans, applesauce, canned tomatoes, curry paste, guacamole, miso, sambal, vinegar, and tahini. Various vegan-friendly sweeteners, you can use include stevia, date syrup, coconut syrup, maple syrup, rice syrup, molasses, organic cane sugar, and agave syrup. Other miscellaneous ingredients include trail mix, coffee, cocoa, baking powder, cornstarch, tea, and potato starch.

Vegan Dairy Alternatives

These days, there are plenty of dairy alternatives available. Various plant-based dairy alternatives you can choose from include soymilk, hemp milk, flax milk, coconut milk, almond milk, rice milk, and cashew milk. Apart from this, you can also include almond yogurt, coconut yogurt, soy yogurt, and any other soy products like tofu and tempeh.

While shopping, ensure that you always read through the list of ingredients present on the product you want to purchase. Also, any product that is rich in saturated fats must be avoided. Whenever buying any processed foods, always opt for organic varieties.

Start with what you as of today have on your kitchen and clean area. If that you are feeling overpowered, begin with a few different vegetables, grains, herbs and flavors, dried organic goods, seeds and nuts, berries and routine meals are grown on the floor. After a time, add new items to your menu. Provided that you will have accumulated the larger part of these things beneath or may have at any speed tried all of them.

As of now in a café? Ask as To if they own a veggie fan menu.

Make Sure You indicate you would like a Dinner free of monster items. Regularly folks do not have the foggiest notion what veggie enthusiast or plant-based approaches and you'll probably end up using milk or cheddar in your plate.

Try to not be timid about creating Your own dish out of the ingredients from the menu. Many eateries should be pleased to support you.

Eat until you consume it. Once in the Café, you'll be able to organize a serving of greens or even a bowl of vegetable soup. Every eatery should, at any rate, have one of these 2 things.

Cultural cafés are in each situation Fantastic options for finding veggie enthusiasts or vegetarian dinners. You can at any speed get vegetables and rice. Create a point to ask the culinary pros forget about all of the oil and salt, on the off possibility they can.

Serving of mixed greens Smorgasbords can be ample. Keep this simple plate guideline: 1/2 non-bland veggies (primitive and cooked), 1/4 whole grains and dull veggies and 1/4 protein (seeds, nuts, vegetables).

On the off possibility that there's No whole nourishment dressing in the plate of mixed greens pub, use vegetable noodle soup, veggie curry or merely lemon peel. This is going to support you with starting to admit slimmer alternatives too.

A Couple of eateries Provide macrobiotic Options, for example a dish cooked with no salt and oils, simply lean and straightforward whole nourishments. I've had the choice to discover a couple of lunch areas in this way in Barcelona.

If you Realize the protein some section of the feast will be more pliable, solicit them to substitute a few from the protein together with veggies, whole grains, nuts/seeds or avocados.

Pastries look yummy at cafés However it is generally better to skirt the desserts. They're commonly high fat and fatty vessels. There are specific cases and a couple of spots provide primitive candies such as chia-pudding or nutty snacks without added sugar and oils.

Constantly be affable and cordial towards café staff and your sidekicks. In the event you're fine to them, everything considered, they will be acceptable for you.

Constantly be appreciative after that the team has qualified your requirements.

Purchase a Juicer or even a Blender on a Plant-Based Diet?

Investigating a juicer that the primary Thing that appeared and caught my attention was clearly the price. They aren't modest. Whatever the situation, buying a fire pit to cook steaks on is not a fryer to get fricasseeing, therefore I put this to the side. The cost actually does not create a difference in the event you're doing so to your wellbeing. Only saying.

The most effective method to Create a Plant-Based Kitchen You Love

Here are a few hints to make a plant-based kitchen you love.

Put things in place

The kitchen will be a room you invest a great deal of energy in, it ought to be satisfying to your eye and make you feel good and cheerful. Paint your kitchen with an upbeat shading. Enhance the dividers with prints, photographs and motivational plaques.

Allow it to stream

You might not have a ton of state about the design of your kitchen particularly things like where the stove and fridge are or how much counter space you have. In any case, you can take advantage of what you need to make a workspace that is productive and utilitarian. On the off chance that you don't have a lot of cupboards for pots and dish, consider hanging a pot rack. Contingent upon the room, it tends to be in the kitchen over the island or against a divider. In my first modest kitchen, my better half balanced a bar in the little open entryway of the kitchen and I hung my pots and skillet from snares. It was space-sparing as well as it made a truly cool gateway. In the event that you don't have a ton of counter space, purchase a major cutting board and spot it over the sink while cooking. Attempt to have your cutting board close to the stove so you can hack and drop. Keep the cooking utensils, oils, vinegar and different things you utilize most close to your work zone or stove for simple reach. Drape your flavors on the divider or get attractive zest holders to hold tight the ice chest. It's simpler to cook while all that you need is close by.

Be Organized

Cooking is significantly increasingly fun when you don't sit around looking for fixing or utensils. Arrange your storeroom things in gatherings. Keep every one of your flavors in a single spot, every one of your grains and beans in another, and every one of your containers, jars and jugs in another. Get clear containers for your grains, beans and vegetables and print names on them. I like to keep all my heating supplies like flours, preparing powder and sugars assembled. Have all your heating dishes in one spot. On the off chance that you don't have bureau space, get a bin to hold them. Keep your veggie lover cookbooks on a rack in the kitchen for motivation and snappy reference. Additionally, hold a note pad to write down your very own thoughts for plans or your shopping list.

The Food

When you have your kitchen set up the manner in which you need it, it's a great opportunity to fill the storeroom and ice chest with all that you have to make astonishing plant-based dishes.

Instruments of the Trade

You will need to have a Dutch Oven pot for stews and bean stews, an enormous pot to cook pasta in, a medium and little pan with covers for cooking grains, sauces and flavors, and 8-inch and 10-inch skillets for pan-sears, sautés and sautéing veggie burgers. You will need a couple of huge preparing sheets for simmering vegetables and a meat dish that can go in the broiler. Regardless of whether you don't prepare a lot, you will likely need a biscuit tin, an 8-inch square brownie skillet, a rectangular portion search for gold or veggie lover meat portion and two 9-inch round cake dish. The most significant devices in any kitchen are the blades. Put resources into a decent culinary expert's blade, a bread blade and a paring blade. Get a couple of vegetable peelers with different sharp edges that cut in various shapes, a grater and a zester. With these fundamental instruments, you will have the option to make a million mind-blowing plant-based dishes.

Chapter 5: What to Eat and What to Avoid

Foods to Avoid on the Vegan Diet

On a vegan diet, you should avoid consuming any animal foods or foods that contain ingredients that were derived from animals. The list of foods to avoid on a vegan diet include: • Poultry and meat. This includes organic meat, wild meat, chicken, turkey, duck, quail, beef, lamb, pork, veal, *etc.*

- Eggs. This can be from any animals including chickens, fish, ostriches, *etc.*

- Seafood and fish. This includes all types of fish and seafood including shrimp, squid, crab, lobster, mussels, anchovies, scallops, *etc.*

- Dairy products. This includes cheese, butter, cream, yogurt, milk, *etc.*

- Bee products. This includes honey, royal jelly, bee pollen, *etc.*

- Animal-based products. This list includes fish derived omega-3 fatty acids, animal derived vitamin D3, whey, lactose, egg white albumen, gelatin, shellac L-cysteine, casein, *etc.*

This list is pretty extensive but there are still some surprising foods that you may not realize are not vegan friendly. This list includes:

- Milk chocolate. Cocoa itself is vegan but milk, milk products, whey, and casein are often added to chocolate.

- Wine and beer. A gelatin-based substance which is derived from fish is often used as a clarifying agent in the manufacture of wine and beer.

- Sugar. Table sugar, which is made from sugar beets or sugarcane, is both completely fine to use. However, some sugars are processed with bone char, which is used in the refining process to help whiten sugar. Bone char is not vegan-friendly.

- Sugary snacks. Some of your favorite candies like gummies and marshmallows contain gelatin, which is derived from animals, and hence not vegan-friendly.

- Red processed foods. Some foods such as yogurt, fruit juices, soda, and candy contain an ingredient called carmine (otherwise known as red dye), which is derived from an insect.

- Non-dairy creamers. Some of these contain a milk-based derivative called sodium caseinate.

- Worcestershire sauce. Traditional recipes for this include anchovies. Note that there are vegan-friendly options available.

- Bread. Many common bread options include egg, butter, milk and other animal byproducts in the ingredient list. Luckily, there are bread recipes available which do not contain such ingredients.

- Omega-3 fortified products. Ensure that the packaging for your omega-3 fortified purchases do not contain fish-based ingredients like sardines, anchovies, and tilapia.

Foods to Eat on the Vegan Diet

This list includes plant and plant-based products such as:

- Fruits and vegetables

- Whole grains, cereals, and pseudo-cereals such as spelt, quinoa, and teff—all of which are high-protein options that are also great sources of complex carbs, B vitamins, and several minerals such as zinc, iron, potassium, to name a few, and fiber.

- Fermented and sprouted plant foods. This includes pickles, kimchi, Ezekiel bread, miso, natto, and tempeh.

- Nutritional yeast. This is a great protein supplement you can include in dishes as a substitute for cheese given its cheesy flavor.

- Seeds such as chia seeds, flax seeds, and hemp seeds which are good sources of protein and omega-3 fatty acids.

- Nuts and nut butters are great sources of fiber, magnesium, zinc, selenium, vitamin E, and iron. The unroasted and unblanched varieties are best.

- Legumes such as lentils, beans, and peas are great protein sources and increase nutrient absorption.

- Plant-based protein replacements. This includes tofu, tempeh, and seitan. They make great replacements for meat, fish, poultry, and eggs in recipes.

- Calcium-fortified plant milks and yogurts. These are a great replacement for milk and yogurt and help provide the recommended daily supplement of calcium. Try to get versions that have been fortified with vitamin B12 and D when possible.

Some vegans we find it difficult to ensure that they get adequate supplies of all nutrients required daily.

Therefore, supplements can be taken to fortify the vegan diet. Supplements include EPA and DHA, which are omega-3 fatty acids which can be sourced from algae oil, Iron, vitamin D, vitamin B12, calcium, zinc and iodine, which can also be supplemented by adding 1/2 teaspoon of iodized salt to your diet.

Eating Out on a Vegan Diet

Eating out on any diet can be challenging and the same can be said for eating out as a vegan. The way to make this as stress-free as possible for you is to plan ahead. To make this process easier for you, here are a few tips that you can employ while eating out:

- Try to find the restaurant menu online beforehand so that you can determine if there are any vegan options available.

- You may try calling ahead to arrange a special vegan dish with the chef.

- At the restaurants, you can simply ask the staff about any vegan options available before you get seated so that you can know if this restaurant is the right choice for you.

- Try ethnic restaurants such as Mexican, Thai, Indian, Middle-Eastern, and Ethiopian cuisine because they tend to have several natural vegan-friendly options.

- At a restaurant, try to identify the vegetarian options on the menu and ask if any dairy or egg products can be removed to make the dish vegan-friendly.

- If there are no vegan meal options, order several vegan appetizers or side dishes to make up a meal.

Also check out the new vegetarian and vegan restaurants within your neighborhood. With the widespread awareness of leading a plant-based lifestyle gaining traction each day, there are always newer pure vegan and vegetarian restaurants also popping up everywhere you go!

Chapter 6: Eating Healthy and Losing Weight

Eat healthily and lose weight together. Being overweight is a common problem today and we see many people trying to lose weight. They try diets, bodybuilding and training camps, but somehow they often do not succeed in the long term.

A key aspect of losing weight is controlling your eating habits. If you have been replacing fast food with healthy food since childhood, it is complicated to make permanent changes. Start with some minor changes that will allow you to practice eating healthy delicious foods.

Only when you have strong interest in losing weight will you make the compromises necessary. With proper exercise and healthy food, you can lose weight.

As a vegan, you are automatically put in an all plant-based diet whether you are trying to lose weight or not.

Guides that talk about a specific vegan diet to lose weight or two can help you stay on track, but as a vegan you don't need one. In a lifestyle of ingredient label readings and exercise, every day you're already working on losing or maintaining your body weight.

Following these steps below will help you to eat healthily, shed pounds at a rapid pace.

Start each day with a good dose of protein

If you want to burn more calories and lose weight faster, protein is the nutrient for you. Not only is it the building block of muscle tissue which helps to keep your metabolism running strong, protein is also a thermogenic food, meaning that its digestion requires a lot of calories from the body. When you eat protein, the calorie burn rate of your body rises. Great for weight loss. Lean protein is best, which is why I start the day with eggs.

Eat lots of fiber

Perfect to curb your appetite and give you that full feeling for hours, fiber is vital for calorie control and sensible eating. It's good for the digestion, high to reduce hunger, simply excellent for weight loss. It is also healthy for your entire digestive system.

Fruit and vegetables

What better way to reduce cravings for sweets than to eat some fruit and vegetables? Rich in vitamins, antioxidants, fiber, and a host of other goodies, a good variety of fruit and vegetables is key for healthy eating and long term weight loss.

Nuts and seeds

¼ great source of good fats, protein, and a merely excellent way to add flavor and crunchiness to nearly every dish. Nuts and almonds are rich in calories and so should be eaten in moderation. However, they are so good for you that you should have some every single day. I often eat them as snacks or sprinkle them on my salad.

Water

While water isn't a food, I have to mention it here because it's crucial for good health and weight loss. Drinking water is part of eating healthy. Water helps purify your body, improves internal bodily function, eases waste elimination, reduces hunger, and many more things that are merely crucial for you. Drink at least 8 glasses of water every day.

Transitioning to the Vegan Diet

For those new to vegan diets, the idea of suddenly refusing to eat meat and dairy products can be quite scary. In today's society, most people put meat, dairy, and eggs in a large percentage of their daily food. Therefore, if you are interested in a vegan diet and are tired of spending the night with your favorite foods, you should make a gradual transition to a vegan diet.

Chapter 7: A Complete 30 days Diet Meal Plan, day by day

Week 1: Meal Plan

Monday

Breakfast: Green Kick start Smoothie

Lunch: Herby Giant Couscous with Asparagus and Lemon

Dinner: Baked Root Veg with Chili

Tuesday

Breakfast: Apple Pie Breakfast Farro

Lunch: Veggieful' Chili

Dinner: Autumn Stuffed Enchiladas

Wednesday

Breakfast: Banana Bread Rice Pudding

Lunch: Red Curry Lentils

Dinner: Creamy Vegetable Casserole

Thursday

Breakfast: Apple and cinnamon oatmeal

Lunch: Black-Bean Veggie Burritos

Dinner: Butternut Squash Alfredo

Friday

Breakfast: Spiced orange breakfast couscous

Lunch: Baked Red Bell Peppers

Dinner: Vegan Lasagna

Saturday

Breakfast: Breakfast parfaits

Lunch: Quick Quinoa Casserole

Dinner: Creamy, Dreamy Dahl

Sunday

Breakfast: Sweet potato and kale hash

Lunch: Mexican Casserole

Dinner: Easy Thai Coconut Curry

Week 2: Meal Plan

Monday

Breakfast: Delicious Oat Meal

Lunch: Vegan Mac and Cheese

Dinner: Sabrosa Spanish Paella

Tuesday

Breakfast: Breakfast Cherry Delight

Lunch: Mushroom Ragout

Dinner: Vegan Festive Nut Roast

Wednesday

Breakfast: Crazy Maple and Pear Breakfast

Lunch: Pumpkin Pilaf

Dinner: Roasted Vegetable Pie

Thursday

Breakfast: Hearty French Toast Bowls

Lunch: Herby Giant Couscous with Asparagus and Lemon

Dinner: Epic Vegan Holiday Roast

Friday

Breakfast: Tofu Burrito

Lunch: Veggieful' Chili

Dinner: Baked Root Veg with Chili

Saturday

Breakfast: Tasty Mexican Breakfast

Lunch: Red Curry Lentils

Dinner: Autumn Stuffed Enchiladas

Sunday

Breakfast: Green Kick start Smoothie

Lunch: Black-Bean Veggie Burritos

Dinner: Creamy Vegetable Casserole

Week 3: Meal Plan

Monday

Breakfast: Warm Quinoa Breakfast Bowl

Lunch: Baked Red Bell Peppers

Dinner: Butternut Squash Alfredo

Tuesday

Breakfast: Banana Bread Rice Pudding

Lunch: Quick Quinoa Casserole

Dinner: Vegan Lasagna

Wednesday

Breakfast: Apple and cinnamon oatmeal

Lunch: Mexican Casserole

Dinner: Creamy, Dreamy Dahl

Thursday

Breakfast: Spiced orange breakfast couscous

Lunch: Vegan Mac and Cheese

Dinner: Butternut Squash Alfredo

Friday

Breakfast: Breakfast parfaits

Lunch: Mushroom Ragout

Dinner: Vegan Lasagna

Saturday

Breakfast: Sweet potato and kale hash

Lunch: Herby Giant Couscous with Asparagus and Lemon

Dinner: Easy Thai Coconut Curry

Sunday

Breakfast: Delicious Oat Meal

Lunch: Pumpkin Pilaf

Dinner: Broccoli & Walnut Pesto

Week 4: Meal plan

Monday

Breakfast: Breakfast Cherry Delight

Lunch: Baked Red Bell Peppers

Dinner: Vegan Festive Nut Roast

Tuesday

Breakfast: Crazy Maple and Pear Breakfast

Lunch: Herby Giant Couscous with Asparagus and Lemon

Dinner: Roasted Vegetable Pie

Wednesday

Breakfast: Veggieful' Chili

Lunch: Colcannon-Topped Vegan Shepherds' Pie

Dinner: Easy Thai Coconut Curry

Thursday

Breakfast: Tofu Burrito

Lunch: Baked Red Bell Peppers

Dinner: Vegan Festive Nut Roast

Friday

Breakfast: Tasty Mexican Breakfast

Lunch: Vegan Mac and Cheese

Dinner: Sabrosa Spanish Paella

Saturday

Breakfast: Sweet potato and kale hash

Lunch: Pumpkin Pilaf

Dinner: Butternut Squash Alfredo

Sunday

Breakfast: Delicious Oat Meal

Lunch: Quick Quinoa Casserole

Dinner: Roasted Vegetable Pie

Chapter 8: Basic Shopping list

Asparagus

Avocados

Baby carrots (e.g. Chantenay)

Handful baby spinach

large carrot small baby carrots

Cherry tomatoes

Curly kale

Fresh basil

Fresh coriander

Lemons

Lime

Mixed mushrooms

Onions

Baking potatoes

Red onions

Romano peppers

Shallots mon

Spring onions

Sweet potato

Borlotti beans (tinned)

Brazil nuts

Tin cannellini beans

Cashew nuts

Tin chickpeas

Tin chopped tomatoes

Gnocchi (ready-made, check it is vegan)

Tin green or brown lentils

Microwave packet brown basmati rice

Passata

Roasted red pepper (from a jar)

Spelt spaghetti (or normal wheat spaghetti would be fine too)

Sultanas Tue

Tinned black beans

Whole-wheat giant couscous

Coconut yoghurt

Dairy-free cream (soya or oat cream)

Vegan parmesan-style 'cheese'

Vegan sausages

Peas (fresh or frozen)

Vegetables and pulses (e.g. bag frozen Chickpea & Spinach mix with lentils and spinach)

Chapter 9: Breakfast Recipes

Green Kick start Smoothie

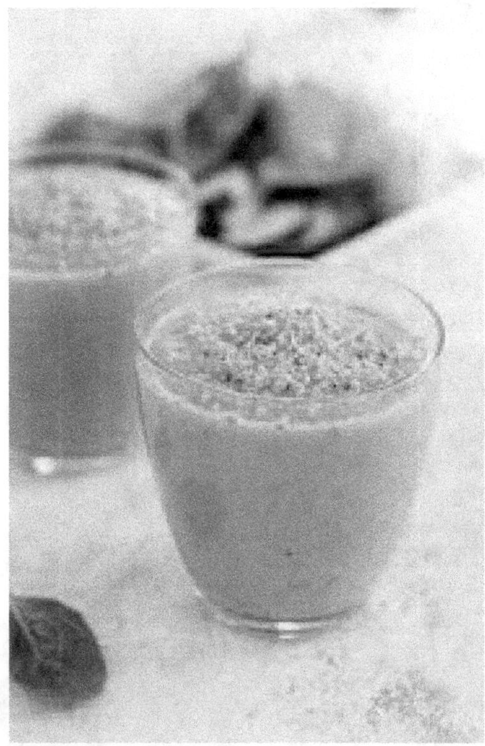

Preparation time: 5 minutes

Servings: 1

Ingredients

- ½ Avocado or 1 banana
- ½ Cup chopped cucumber, peeled if desired
- 1 handful fresh spinach or chopped lettuce
- 1 pear or apple, peeled and cored, or 1 cup unsweetened applesauce
- 2 tablespoons freshly squeezed lime juice
- 1 cup water or nondairy milk, plus more as needed

Additions

- ½-Inch piece peeled fresh ginger
- 1 tablespoon ground flaxseed or chia seeds
- ½ Cup soy yogurt or 3 ounces silken tofu
- Coconut water to replace some of the liquid
- 2 tablespoons chopped fresh mint or ½ cup chopped mango

Directions:

1. In a blender, combine the avocado, cucumber, spinach, pear, lime juice, and water.

2. Add any Additions Ingredients as desired. Purée until smooth and creamy, about 50 seconds. Add

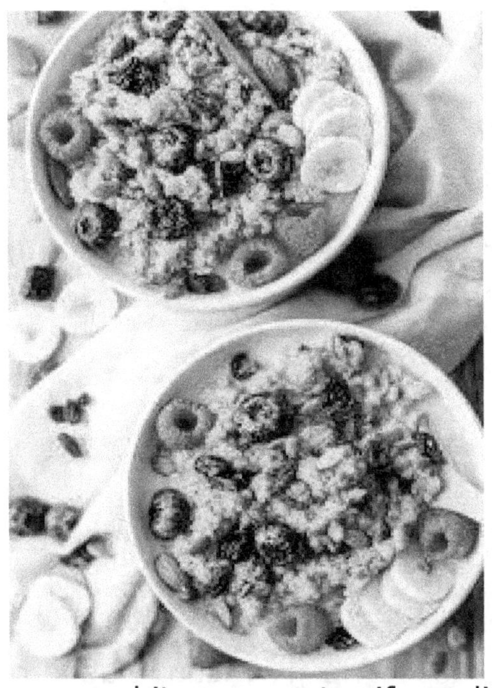

a bit more water if you like a thinner smoothie.

Nutrition: calories: 263; protein: 4g; total fat: 14g; saturated fat: 2g; carbohydrates: 36g; fiber: 10g

Warm Quinoa Breakfast Bowl

Preparation time: 5 minutes

Cooking time: 0 minutes Servings: 4

Ingredients

- 3 cups freshly cooked quinoa
- 1⅓ cups unsweetened soy or almond milk
- 2 bananas, sliced
- 1 cup raspberries
- 1 cup blueberries
- ½ Cup chopped raw walnuts
- ¼ Cup maple syrup

Directions:

1. Divide the Ingredients among 4 bowls, starting with a base of ¾ cup quinoa, ⅓ cup milk, ½ banana, ¼ cup raspberries, ¼ cup blueberries, and 2 tablespoons walnuts.
2. Drizzle 1 tablespoon of maple syrup over the top of each bowl.

Banana Bread Rice Pudding

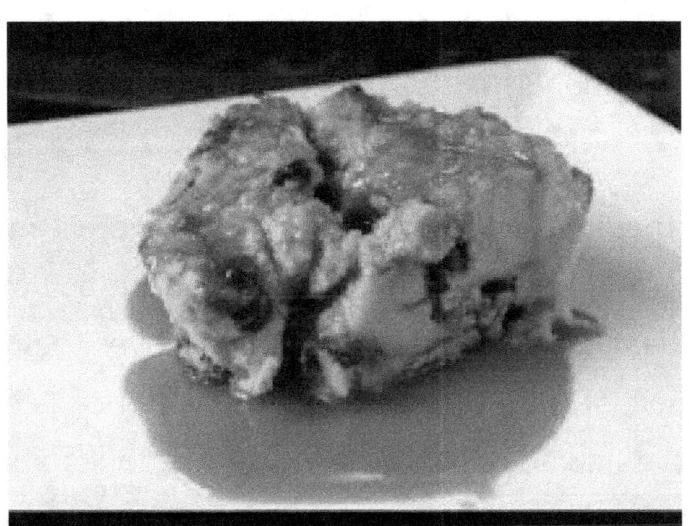

Preparation time: 5 minutes

Cooking time: 50 minutes Servings: 4

Ingredients

- 1cup brown rice
- 1½ cups water
- 1½ cups nondairy milk
- 3 tablespoons sugar (omit if using a sweetened nondairy milk)
- 2 teaspoons pumpkin pie spice or ground cinnamon

- 2 bananas
- 3 tablespoons chopped walnuts or sunflower seeds (optional)

Directions

1. In a medium pot, combine the rice, water, milk, sugar, and pumpkin pie spice. Bring to a boil over high heat, turn the heat to low, and cover the pot. Simmer, stirring occasionally, until the rice is soft and the liquid is absorbed. White rice takes about 20 minutes; brown rice takes about 50 minutes.
2. Smash the bananas and stir them into the cooked rice. Serve topped with walnuts (if using). Leftovers will keep refrigerated in an airtight container for up to 5 days.

Nutrition: calories: 479; protein: 9g; total fat: 13g; saturated fat: 1g; carbohydrates: 86g; fiber: 7g

Apple and cinnamon oatmeal

Preparation time: 10 minutes

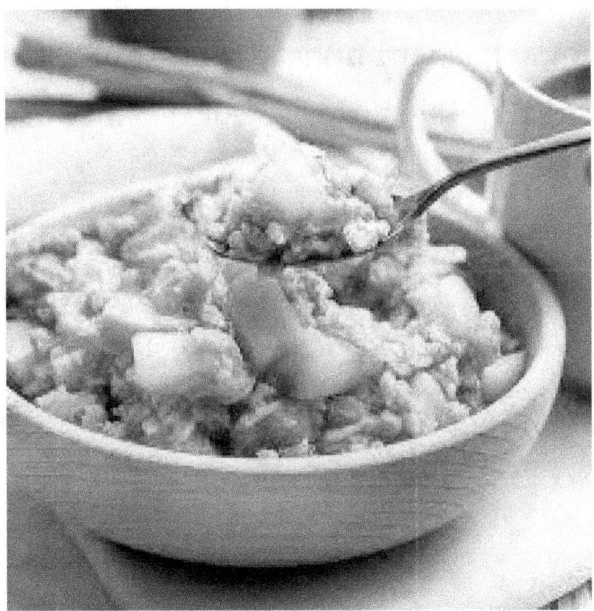

Cooking time:10 minutes Servings: 2

Ingredients

- 1¼ cups apple cider
- 1 apple, peeled, cored, and chopped
- ⅔ Cup rolled oats

- 1 teaspoon ground cinnamon
- 1 tablespoon pure maple syrup or agave (optional)

Directions

1. In a medium saucepan, bring the apple cider to a boil over medium-high heat. Stir in the apple, oats, and cinnamon.
2. Bring the cereal to a boil and turn down heat to low. Simmer until the oatmeal thickens, 3 to 4 minutes. Spoon into two bowls and sweeten with maple syrup, if using. Serve hot.

Spiced orange breakfast couscous

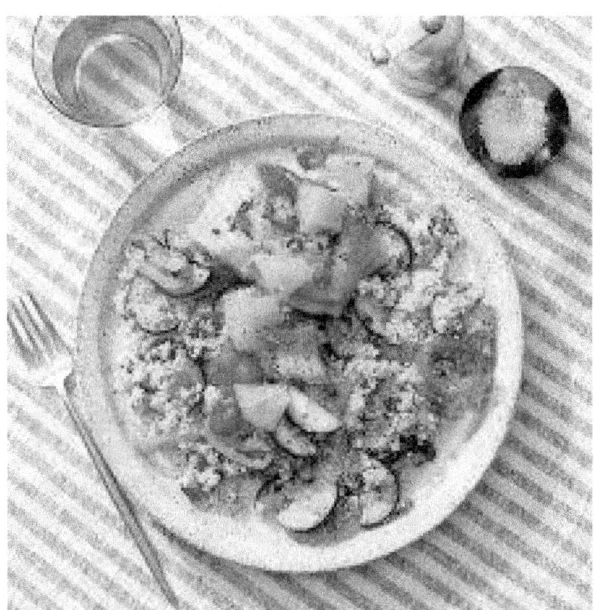

Preparation time: 10 minutes

Cooking time: 10 minutes Servings: 4

Ingredients

- 3 cups orange juice
- 1½ cups couscous
- 1 teaspoon ground cinnamon
- ¼ Teaspoon ground cloves
- ½ Cup dried fruit, such as raisins or apricots
- ½ Cup chopped almonds or other nuts or seeds

Directions

1. In a small saucepan, bring the orange juice to a boil. Add the couscous, cinnamon, and cloves and remove from heat. Cover the pan with a lid and allow to sit until the -couscous softens, about 5 minutes.
2. Fluff the couscous with a fork and stir in the dried fruit and nuts. Serve -immediately.

Nutrition: calories 120, fat 1, fiber 2, carbs 3, protein 5

Breakfast parfaits

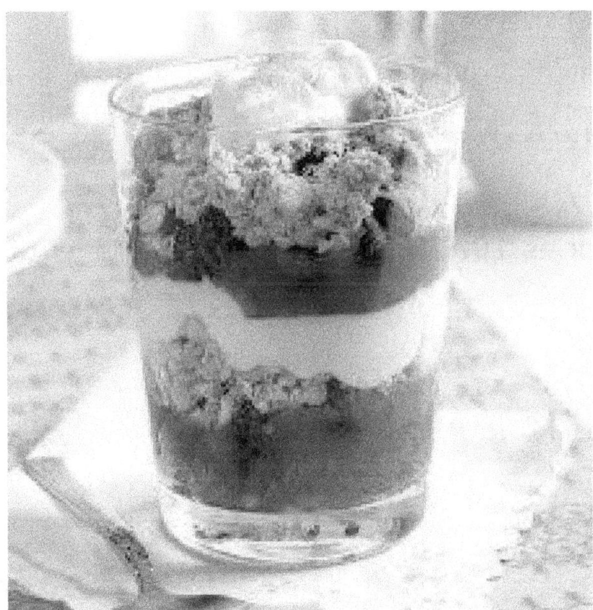

Preparation time: 15 minutes

Cooking time: 0 minutes Servings: 2

Ingredients

- One 14-ounce can coconut milk, refrigerated overnight
- 1 cup granola
- ½ Cup walnuts
- 1 cup sliced strawberries or other seasonal berries

Directions

1. Pour off the canned coconut-milk liquid and retain the solids.
2. In two parfait glasses, layer the coconut-milk solids, granola, walnuts, and -strawberries. Serve immediately.

Nutrition: calories 100, fat 1, fiber 2, carbs 3, protein 5

Sweet potato and kale hash

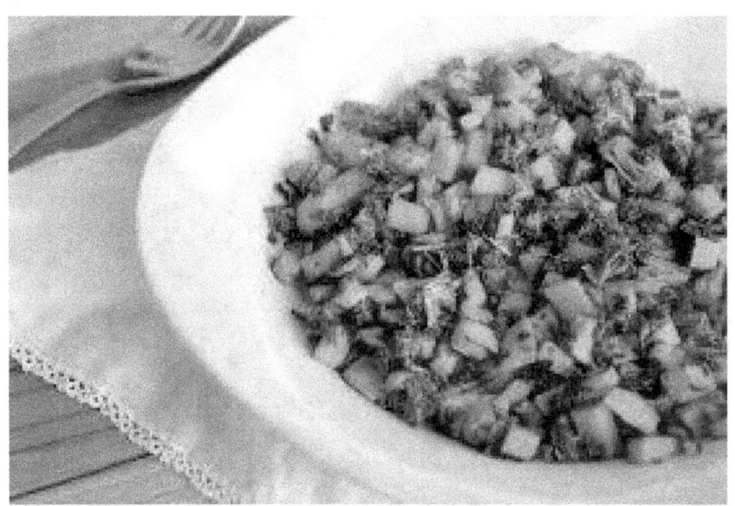

Preparation time: 10 minutes

Cooking time: 15 minutes Servings: 2

Ingredients

- 1 sweet potato
- 2 tablespoons olive oil
- ½ Onion, chopped
- 1 carrot, peeled and chopped
- 2 garlic cloves, minced
- ½ Teaspoon dried thyme
- 1 cup chopped kale
- Sea salt

- Freshly ground black pepper

Directions

1. Prick the sweet potato with a fork and microwave on high until soft, about 5 minutes. Remove from the microwave and cut into ¼-inch cubes.
2. In a large nonstick sauté pan, heat the olive oil over medium-high heat. Add the onion and carrot and cook until softened, about 5 minutes. Add the garlic and thyme and cook until the garlic is fragrant, about 30 seconds.
3. Add the sweet potatoes and cook until the potatoes begin to brown, about 7 -minutes. Add the kale and cook just until it wilts, 1 to 2 minutes. Season with salt and pepper. Serve immediately.

Nutrition: calories 90, fat 1, fiber 2, carbs 3, protein 5

Delicious Oat Meal

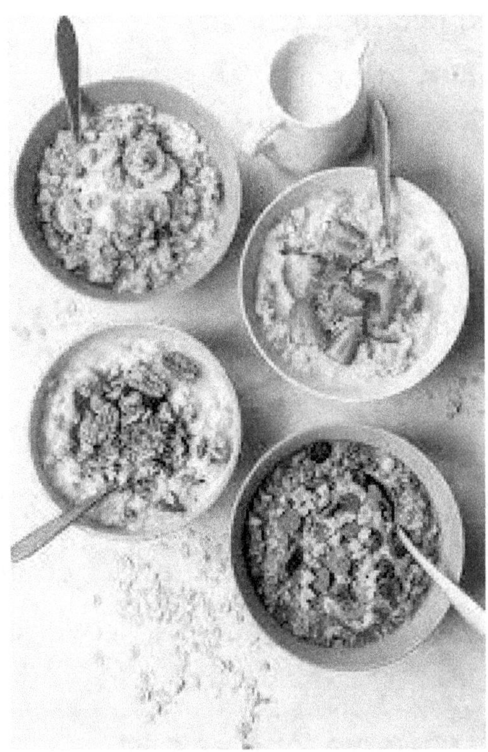

Preparation time: 10 minutes

Cooking time: 6 hours

Servings: 4

Ingredients:

- 3 cups water
- 3 cups almond milk

- 1 and ½ cups steel oats
- 4 dates, pitted and chopped
- 1 teaspoon cinnamon, ground
- 2 tablespoons coconut sugar
- ½ Teaspoon ginger powder
- A pinch of nutmeg, ground
- A pinch of cloves, ground
- 1 teaspoon vanilla extract

Directions:

1. Put water and milk in your slow cooker and stir.
2. Add oats, dates, cinnamon, sugar, ginger, nutmeg, cloves and vanilla extract, stir, cover and cook on low for 6 hours.
3. Divide into bowls and serve for breakfast.
4. Enjoy!

Nutrition: calories 120, fat 1, fiber 2, carbs 3, protein 5

Breakfast Cherry Delight

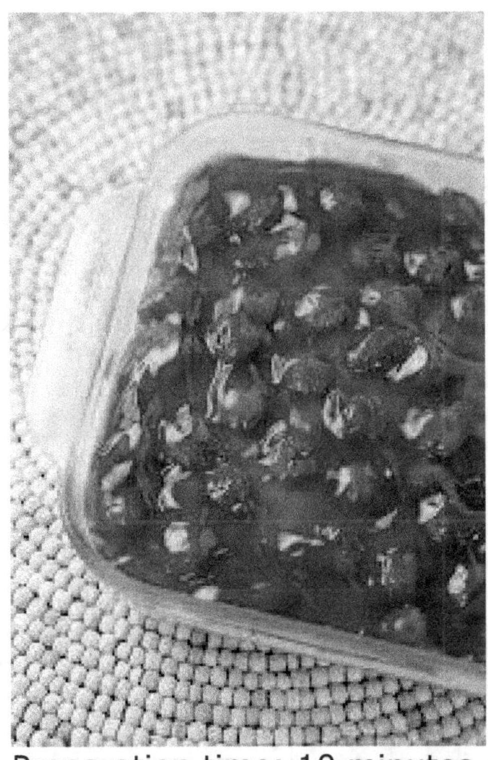

Preparation time: 10 minutes

Cooking time: 8 hours and 10 minutes

Servings: 4

Ingredients:

- 2 cups almond milk
- 2 cups water

- 1 cup steel cut oats
- 2 tablespoons cocoa powder
- 1/3 cup cherries, pitted
- ¼ Cup maple syrup
- ½ Teaspoon almond extract

For the sauce:

- 2 tablespoons water
- 1 and ½ cups cherries, pitted and chopped
- ¼ Teaspoon almond extract

Directions:

1. Put the almond milk in your slow cooker.
2. Add 2 cups water, oats, cocoa powder, 1/3 cup cherries, maples syrup and ½ teaspoon almond extract.
3. Stir, cover and cook on low for 8 hours.
4. In a small pan, mix 2 tablespoons water with 1 and ½ cups cherries and ¼ teaspoon almond

extract, stir well, bring to a simmer over medium heat and cook for 10 minutes until it thickens.

5. Divide oatmeal into breakfast bowls, top with the cherries sauce and serve.

6. Enjoy!

Nutrition: calories 150, fat 1, fiber 2, carbs 6, protein 5

Crazy Maple and Pear Breakfast

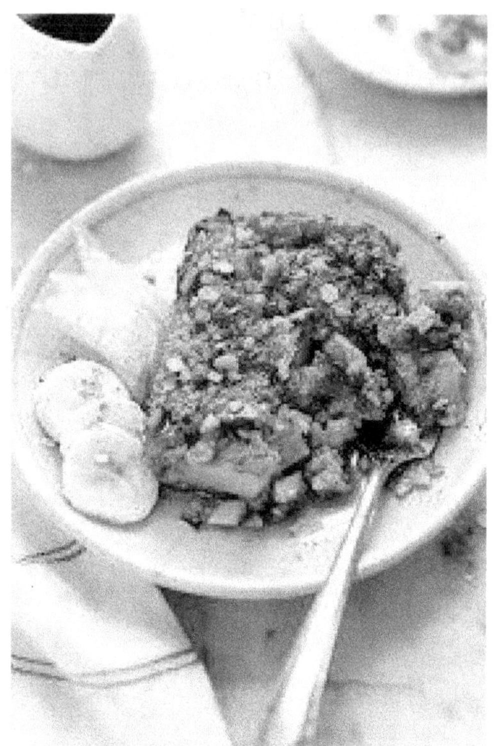

Preparation time: 10 minutes

Cooking time: 9 hours

Servings: 2

Ingredients:

- 1 pear, cored and chopped
- ½ Teaspoon maple extract

- 2 cups coconut milk
- ½ Cup steel cut oats
- ½ Teaspoon vanilla extract
- 1 tablespoon stevia
- ¼ Cup walnuts, chopped for serving
- Cooking spray

Directions:

1. Spray your slow cooker with some cooking spray and add coconut milk.
2. Also, add maple extract, oats, pear, stevia and vanilla extract, stir, cover and cook on low for 9 hours.
3. Stir your oatmeal again, divide it into breakfast bowls and serve with chopped walnuts on top.
4. Enjoy!

Nutrition: calories 150, fat 3, fiber 2, carbs 6, protein 6

Hearty French Toast Bowls

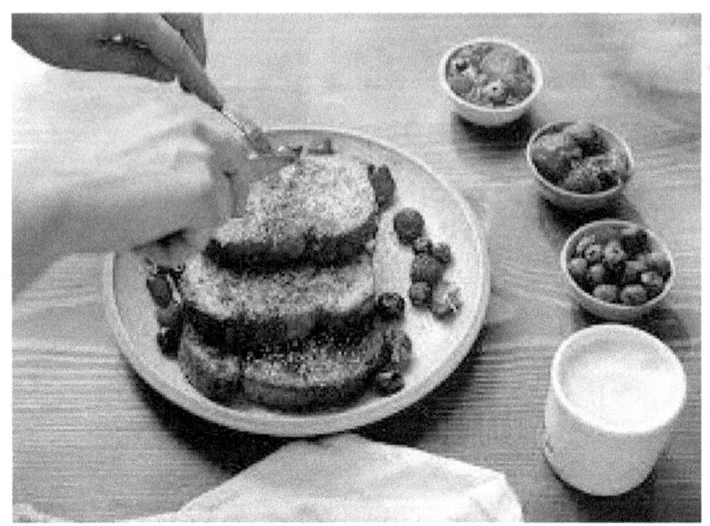

Preparation time: 10 minutes

Cooking time: 5 hours

Servings: 4

Ingredients:

- 1 and ½ cups almond milk
- 1 cup coconut cream
- 1 tablespoon vanilla extract
- ½ Tablespoon cinnamon powder
- 2 tablespoons maple syrup
- ¼ Cup spenda

- 2 apples, cored and cubed
- ½ Cup cranberries, dried
- 1 pound vegan bread, cubed
- Cooking spray

Directions:

1. Spray your slow cooker with some cooking spray and add the bread.
2. Also, add cranberries and apples and stir gently.
3. Add milk, coconut cream, maple syrup, vanilla extract, cinnamon powder and splenda.
4. Stir, cover and cook on low for 5 hours.
5. Divide into bowls and serve right away.
6. Enjoy!

Nutrition: calories 140, fat 2, fiber 3, carbs 6, protein 2

Tofu Burrito

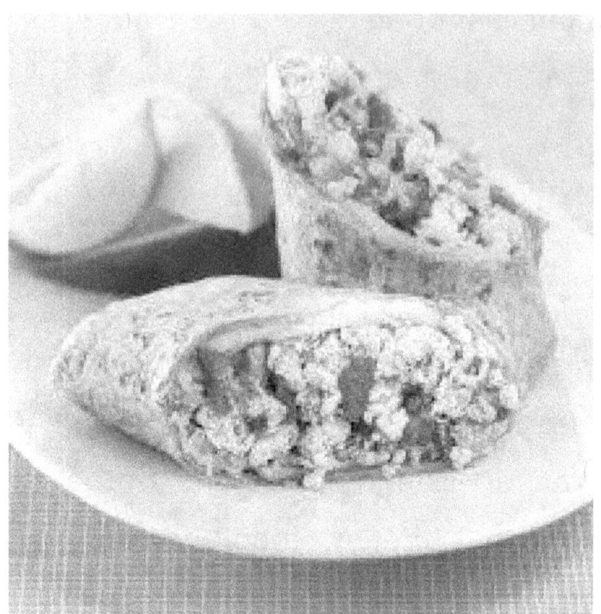

Preparation time: 10 minutes

Cooking time: 8 hours

Servings: 4

Ingredients:

- 15 ounces canned black beans, drained
- 2 tablespoons onions, chopped
- 7 ounces tofu, drained and crumbled
- 2 tablespoons green bell pepper, chopped

- ½ Teaspoon turmeric
- ¾ Cup water
- ¼ Teaspoon smoked paprika
- ¼ Teaspoon cumin, ground
- ¼ Teaspoon chili powder
- A pinch of salt and black pepper
- 4 gluten free whole wheat tortillas
- Avocado, chopped for serving
- Salsa for serving

Directions:

1. Put black beans in your slow cooker.
2. Add onions, tofu, bell pepper, turmeric, water, paprika, cumin, chili powder, a pinch of salt and pepper, stir, cover and cook on low for 8 hours.
3. Divide this on each tortilla, add avocado and salsa, wrap, arrange on plates and serve.
4. Enjoy!

Nutrition: calories 130, fat 4, fiber 2, carbs 5, protein 4

Tasty Mexican Breakfast

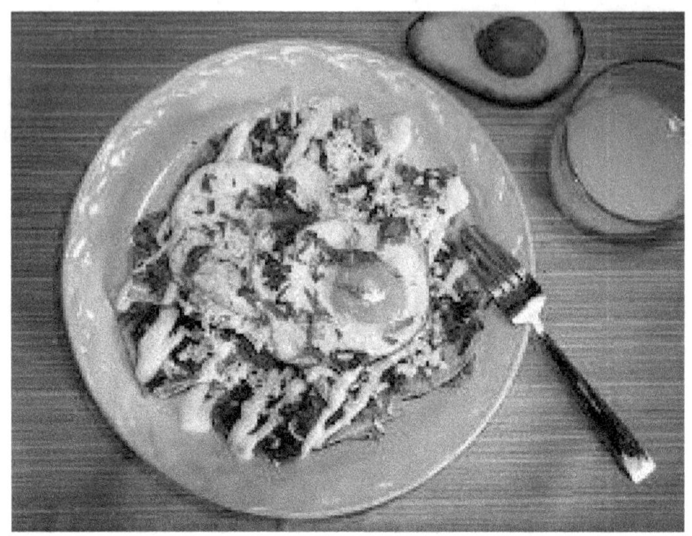

Preparation time: 10 minutes

Cooking time: 2 hours

Servings: 4

Ingredients:

- 1 cup brown rice
- 1 cup onion, chopped
- 2 cups veggie stock
- 1 red bell pepper, chopped
- 1 green bell pepper, chopped
- 4 ounces canned green chilies, chopped

- 15 ounces canned black beans, drained
- A pinch of salt
- Black pepper to the taste

For the salsa:

- 3 tablespoons lime juice
- 1 avocado, pitted, peeled and cubed
- ½ Cup cilantro, chopped
- ½ Cup green onions, chopped
- ½ Cup tomato, chopped
- 1 poblano pepper, chopped
- 2 tablespoons olive oil
- ½ Teaspoon cumin

Directions:

1. Put the stock in your slow cooker.
2. Add rice, onions and beans, stir, cover and cook on high for 1 hour and 30 minutes.

3. Add chilies, red and green bell peppers, a pinch of salt and black pepper, stir, cover again and cook on high for 30 minutes more.

4. Meanwhile, in a bowl, mix avocado with green onions, tomato, poblano pepper, cilantro, oil, cumin, a pinch of salt, black pepper and lime juice and stir really well.

5. Divide rice mix into bowls; top each with the salsa you've just made and serve.

6. Enjoy!

Nutrition: calories 140, fat 2, fiber 2, carbs 5, protein 5

Chapter 10: Lunch Recipes

Herby Giant Couscous with Asparagus and Lemon

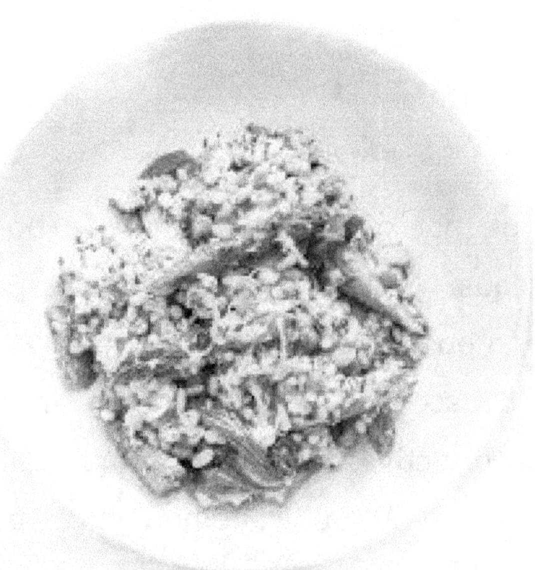

Preparation time: 5 minutes

Servings: 2 Servings

Ingredients

- 150 g giant couscous

- 100 g asparagus tips

- 100 g frozen peas

- 3 tbsp. walnut oil

- Juice and zest of 1 lemon

- Handful fresh parsley

- Handful of fresh mint

- Handful baby spinach

- 2 tbsp. pine nuts

Direction

1. Bring a large pot of salted water to a boil. Add giant couscous. After 5 minutes, add asparagus and peas and boil for another 4 minutes.

2. While the couscous is cooking, cook in a mini blender (or directly in a bowl, sharp knife and elbow grease!), Walnut oil, lemon juice, parsley, and mint.

3. Drain the couscous and immediately stir the dressing of the baby herb and spinach.

4. Divide between two plates and crush with pine nuts and lemon lotion.

Nutrition: calories: 263; protein: 4g; total fat: 14g; saturated fat: 2g; carbohydrates: 36g; fiber: 10g

Veggieful' Chili

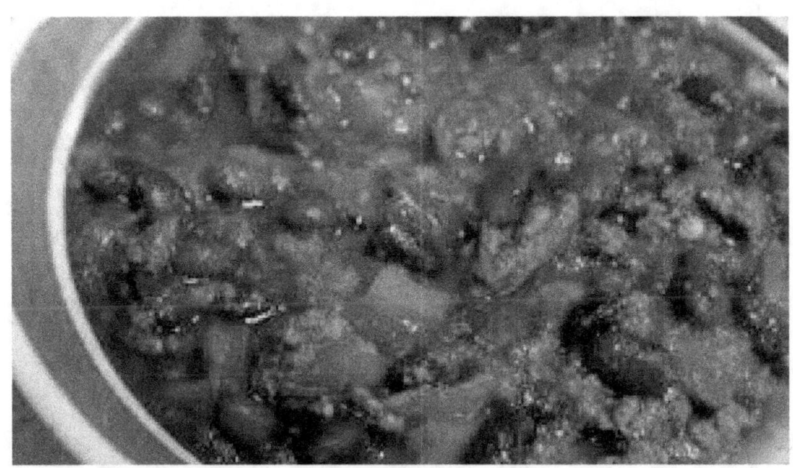

Serves: 8

Preparation Time: 15 minutes

Ingredients :

- 1½ cups raw black beans
- 1½ cups raw kidney beans
- 2 tbsp. olive oil
- 2 red onions (medium, diced)
- 1 clove garlic (minced)

- 2 tsp. cumin

- ¼ tsp. cayenne pepper

- 2 tsp. oregano

- 1 zucchini (medium, diced)

- 1 yellow squash (small, diced)

- 1 red bell pepper (small, diced)

- 2 cups water

- 1 jalapeño (medium, diced)

- 1 cup tomato paste

- 1 (200g) can sweet corn (drained)

- 1 tbsp. chili powder

- Salt and pepper to taste

Directions:

1. Prepare the black and kidney beans according to the Directions.

2. Take a large pan, put it on medium high heat and add the olive oil.

3. Sautee the diced red onions for about 5 minutes.

4. Blend in the garlic, cumin, cayenne pepper, oregano while stirring.

5. Add the diced zucchini, squash, bell pepper and stir again.
6. Allow the mixture to fry for a few minutes while constantly stirring.
7. Lower the heat to medium and add 2 cups of water, jalapeño, tomato paste, corn and cooked beans.
8. Stir well while adding the chili powder, salt and optionally more pepper to taste.
9. Reduce the heat to low, cover the pan and let the chili simmer for about 20 minutes.
10. Add more spices like cumin, oregano, chili powder or cayenne pepper to taste.
11. Serve and enjoy warm or allow the chili to cool down to store it in containers!

Nutrition:

Calories: 256 kcal.

Carbs: 43.6g.

Fat: 4.5gr.

Protein: 13g.

Fiber: 16.8g.

Sugar: 8.5g.

Red Curry Lentils

Serves: 6

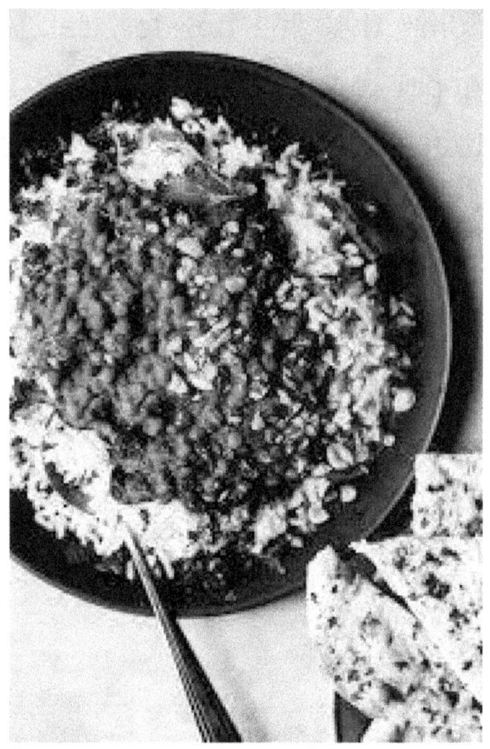

Preparation Time: 20 minutes

Ingredients :

- 1 cup dry red lentils
- 2 tbsp. coconut oil
- 1 tbsp. cumin seeds
- 1 tbsp. coriander seeds
- 8 tomatoes (ripe, cubed)
- 1 head of garlic (chopped or minced)
- 2 tbsp. ginger (chopped)
- 1 tbsp. turmeric
- 1 tsp. cayenne powder
- 3 cups vegetable broth
- 2 tsp. sea salt
- 1 (15oz.) can coconut milk
- ½ cup cherry tomatoes
- ½ cup cilantro (chopped)

Directions:

1. Soak and drain the red lentils according to the Directions but do not cook them yet.
2. Put the coconut oil in a large pot heating over medium high heat.

3. Add the cumin and coriander seeds and garlic. Sauté the Ingredients for about 2 minutes while continuously stirring.
4. Add the freshly cut tomato cubes, ginger, turmeric and a pinch of salt to the pot.
5. Allow the mixture to gently cook, stirring occasionally for 5 minutes.
6. Blend in the red lentils, more salt to taste and cayenne powder.
7. Continue to add 3 cups of vegetable broth to the pot and allow the mixture to come to a soft boil.
8. Reduce the heat to low, cover the pot and allow the dish to simmer for about 30 minutes while stirring occasionally.
9. Once the lentils are soft, add the coconut milk and cherry tomatoes.
10. Bring the mixture back to a simmer before removing it from the heat and stir in the chopped cilantro.
11. Serve warm or allow the curry to cool down before storing.

Nutrition:

Calories: 162 kcal.

Carbs: 19.3g.

Fat: 6.8g.

Protein: 6g.

Fiber: 6.5g.

Sugar: 5.8g.

Black-Bean Veggie Burritos

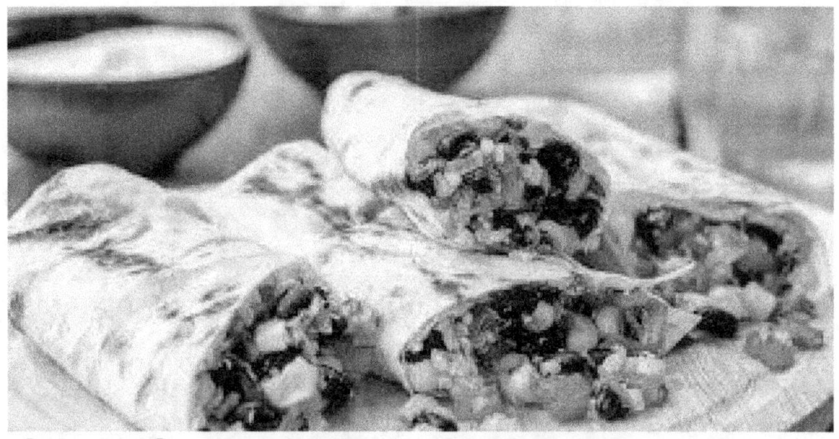

Serves: 8

Preparation Time: 30 minutes

Ingredients

For the filling:

- 2 cups dry black beans
- 1 tbsp. olive oil
- 1 red onion (diced)
- 1 zucchini (cubed)
- 1 red bell pepper (pitted, diced)
- 2 (150g) cans sweet corn (drained, rinsed)
- ¼ cup cilantro (chopped)
- ½ a lime (juiced)
- Salt to taste

For homemade taco seasoning (optional)

- 1 tbsp. chili powder
- 2 tsp. ground cumin
- ½ tsp. paprika powder
- ¼ tsp. of each: garlic powder, onion powder, red pepper flakes, oregano, salt and cayenne
- For the wraps:
- 8 tortilla wraps
- ½ cup no-salt vegan cream cheese
- ½ cup salsa
- 1 cup dry brown rice

Directions:

1. Cook the black beans according to the Directions.

2. Prepare the brown rice according to the recipe.

3. Mix all taco seasoning Ingredients in a bowl and set it aside.

4. Take a large pan, add the olive oil and put it on medium heat.

5. Add the diced red onion. Sauté for 3 minutes while stirring.

6. Add the zucchini and bell pepper and sauté for another 3 minutes.

7. Add in the black beans, corn and the homemade taco seasoning. Stir well and allow the mixture to simmer for about 10 minutes.

8. Turn off the heat and add the cilantro, lime juice and salt to taste.

9. Prepare the burrito by laying out a tortilla wrap and add the filling, salsa, rice and the optional vegan cheese.

10.   Tightly wrap the burrito and place it back in the pan. Heat and press each side for about 2 minutes.

11.   Serve warm or store each tortilla wrapped in aluminum foil in a Ziploc bag.

Nutrition:

Calories: 285 kcal.

Carbs: 40.9g.

Fat: 9.8g.

Protein: 8.6g.

Fiber: 6.7g.

Sugar: 4.3g.

Baked Red Bell Peppers

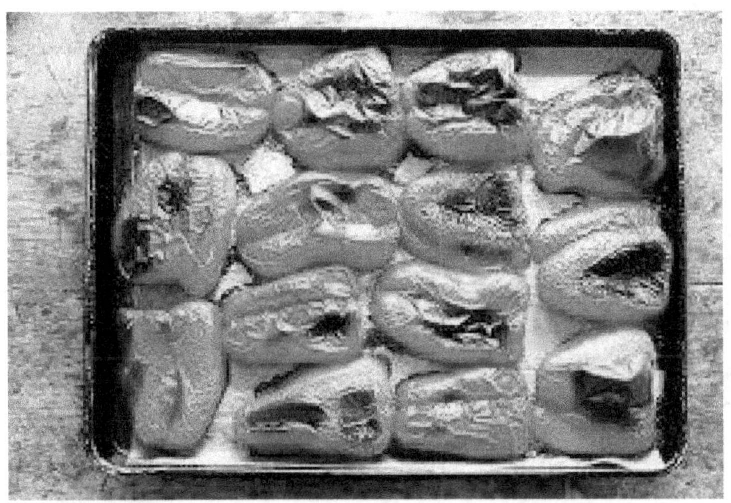

Serves: 8

Preparation Time: 30 minutes

Ingredients :

- 1 cup dry chickpeas
- 1½ cup dry quinoa
- 4 red bell peppers (seeded, halved lengthwise)
- 1½ tbsp. olive oil
- 1 red onion (medium, diced)
- 1 clove garlic (medium, minced)
- 2 tbsp. chili powder
- 2 tsp. cumin
- 1 tsp. cayenne pepper

- 2 tsp. spicy paprika powder
- 2 cups baby spinach (chopped)
- 3 tomatoes (ripe, medium, chopped)
- ¼ cup fresh cilantro (chopped)
- Salt and pepper to taste

Directions:

1. Preheat the oven to 375°F or 190°C.
2. Prepare the chickpeas according to the Directions.
3. Prepare the quinoa according to the recipe.
4. Put the olive oil into a skillet on medium heat.
5. Sautee the diced red onions until soft.
6. Add the garlic, chili powder, cumin, cayenne pepper, paprika powder, salt and pepper to the skillet and stir everything for about 2 minutes.
7. Stir in the remaining Ingredients except the cilantro and add more salt and pepper to taste.
8. Heat the stuffing for another 5 minutes until the Ingredients are browned.
9. Turn off the heat, add dd the cilantro and divide the stuffing into the halved red bell peppers.

10.   Put the peppers on a lightly greased baking tray and cover them with aluminum foil.

11.   Place the tray in the oven for about 20 to 25 minutes.

12.   Take the tray out and allow the bell peppers to sit for about 5 minutes.

13.   Serve right away or allow the stuffed red bell peppers to cool down for storage!

Nutrition:

Calories: 135 kcal.

Carbs: 20g.

Fat: 4g.

Protein: 4.5g.

Fiber: 16.4g.

Sugar: 5.5g.

Quick Quinoa Casserole

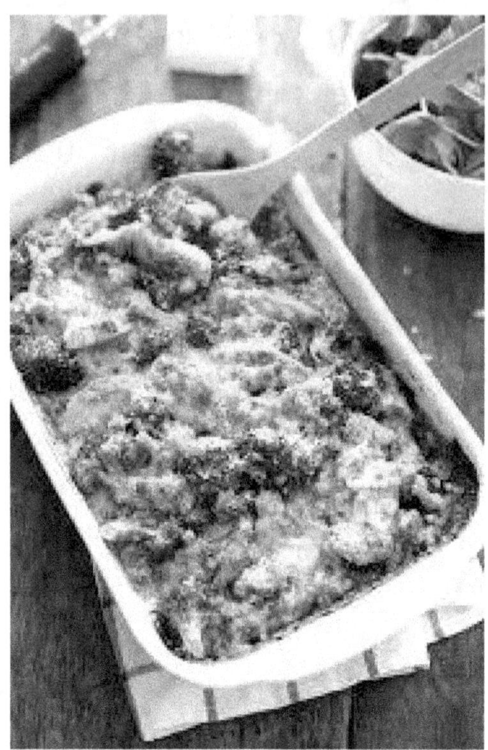

Serves: 9

Preparation Time: 15 minutes

Ingredients :

- 2 cups dry pinto beans
- 1 cup dry quinoa
- 1 (7 oz.) pack tempeh (sliced)
- 2 tbsp. olive oil
- 2 tsp. cumin

- 2 tsp. paprika powder

- 1 cup red onion (diced)

- 2 garlic cloves (minced)

- 6 sweet red peppers (small, sliced)

- 2 (4 oz.) cans green chilies (diced)

- 1 cup Roma tomatoes (diced)

- 2 cups vegetable broth

- Salt and pepper to taste

- ½ cup no-salt cream cheese

- 1 avocado (diced, sliced or mashed)

- ¼ cup green onions (diced)

- ¼ cup cilantro (chopped, fresh)

Directions:

- Cook the pinto beans according to the recipe.

- Put a large skillet greased with the olive oil over medium heat.

- Grill the tempeh slices with a tsp. paprika powder, cumin and salt and pepper to taste for about 5 minutes.

- Take out the grilled tempeh slices and leave it aside.

- Grease the same skillet with olive oil and sauté the onions.
- Add the minced garlic while stirring.
- Blend in the red peppers and stir the Ingredients for about 2 minutes.
- Continue to add the green chilies, cooked pinto beans and quinoa, tomatoes and vegetable broth to the pan along with another tsp. of paprika powder, cumin, salt and pepper to taste.
- Let the mixture cook for about 5 minutes.
- Add the tempeh back to the skillet, stir, cover and reduce the heat to low.
- Cook the mixture for about 15 minutes until the quinoa is soft and most of the broth has been absorbed.
- Remove the skillet from the heat and add vegan cream cheese.
- Put the lid on the skillet and let the dish sit for a minute until the cheese has melted.
- Serve the quick quinoa casserole with fresh avocado slices, green onions and fresh cilantro.
- Enjoy or store!

Nutrition:

Calories: 236 kcal.

Carbs: 24.9g.

Fat: 11g.

Protein: 9.2g.

Fiber: 7.4g.

Sugar: 4g.

Mexican Casserole

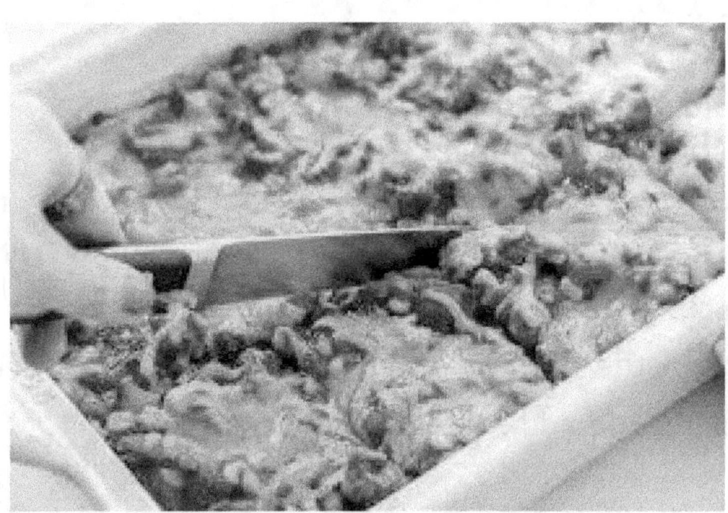

Serves: 4 | Prepping Time: 30 minutes

Ingredients :

- 1 cup dry black beans
- 1 cup dry white beans
- 1 tsp. olive oil
- 3 tbsp. Mexican spice
- 2 cups Mexican salsa
- 1½ cups cashew cheese spread
- 3 bell peppers (red and yellow, chopped)
- 1 red onion (chopped)
- 1 green onion (chopped)
- 1 jalapeno pepper (medium, seeded and chopped)
- Salt and pepper to taste

Directions:

Cook the beans according to the Directions.

1. Preheat oven at 350°F or 175°C.
2. Grease a saucepan with the olive oil. Add Mexican spice, 1 cup of Mexican salsa and stir well.
3. Stir in the cashew cheese, chopped bell peppers, onions and add salt and pepper to taste.

4. Spread ½ cup salsa over the bottom of a casserole dish. Add the beans on top of the salsa and spread out the saucepan mix evenly over the beans.
5. Add the last ½ cup salsa sauce on top and sprinkle some chopped jalapenos on top.
6. Bake the casserole for 15-20 minutes.
7. Enjoy the dish after a short cooling period or let it cool down completely for storing.

Nutrition:

Calories: 442 kcal.

Carbs: 65.9g.

Fat: 11.5g.

Protein: 20.2g.

Fiber: 33.9g.

Sugar: 17.4g.

Vegan Mac and Cheese

Ingredients :

- Cashews (two-thirds cup raw)

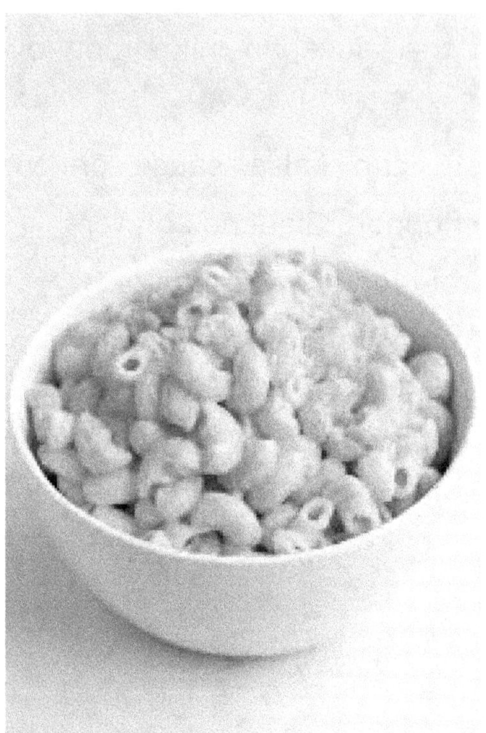

- Chili flakes (quarter teaspoon)

- Nutritional yeast (quarter cup)

- Salt and pepper (to taste)

- Dry mustard powder (half teaspoon)

- Onion powder (half teaspoon)

- Garlic powder (half teaspoon)

- Garlic (three cloves)

- Russet potato (one small)

- White onion (one small)

- Avocado oil (one and a half tablespoons)

- Broccoli (one head)

- Apple cider vinegar (two teaspoons)

- Macaroni (two cups)

Directions:

1. Peel and grate potato and grate. Finely dice the garlic.

2. Heat a large saucepan and oil over medium heat. Put onion and a little salt in the pot and cook until soft.

3. Put the potato, chili flakes and garlic along with mustard, onion and garlic powders into the pot. Stir well until their flavors release, then add one cup of water and the cashews. Keep stirring at a simmer until the potatoes are soft.

4. Pour entire mixture into a blender along with the apple cider vinegar and nutritional yeast, then salt and pepper. The consistency should be that of cheese sauce that is thick yet runny. If it is too

thick, add more water, if it needs more salt or garlic powder, chili flakes or vinegar, do so now according to your taste.

5. Put the pasta on the stove in a large pot with water to cover and a little salt. In another pot, boil the broccoli in bite-sized florets until tender.

6. When both are ready, transfer everything into one pot and cover with the cheese sauce. Combine well, serve and enjoy!

Nutrition: calories: 263; protein: 4g; total fat: 14g; saturated fat: 2g; carbohydrates: 36g; fiber: 10g

Mushroom Ragout

Serves: 10

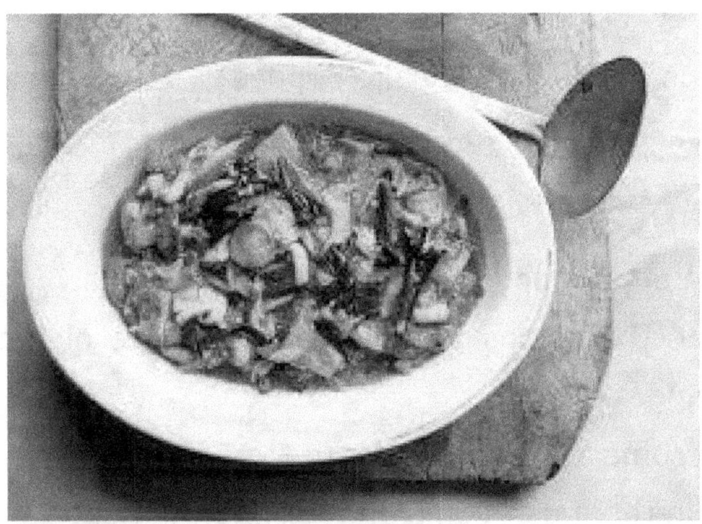

Preparation Time: 45 min |

Ingredients :

- 2 tbsp. olive oil
- 1 sweet onion (large, finely chopped)
- 1 clove garlic (minced)
- 6 cups Portobello mushrooms (chopped)
- ½ cup dry red wine
- 1 cup vegetable broth
- ½ tbsp. nutritional yeast
- ¼ cup basil leaves (chopped)

- ¼ cup no-salt cream cheese substitute with cashew butter
- ¼ cup parsley (optional, chopped)
- Salt and pepper to taste

Directions:

1. Take a large pot and put it on medium heat.
2. Sauté the onions and garlic in the olive oil while stirring.
3. Add some salt and pepper to taste and stir.
4. Mix in the mushrooms and turn up the heat a bit.
5. Cook and stir the mushrooms until most of the liquid in it has evaporated.
6. Add the red wine. Turn the heat up to medium-high and cook the ragout until most of the wine is evaporated.
7. Add the vegetable broth and stir thoroughly.
8. Blend in the nutritional yeast and cook the ragout for about 5 minutes.
9. Add the chopped basil and the no-salt cream cheese.

10.   Lower the heat and keep stirring until the ragout simmers.

11.   Keep stirring occasionally for about 5 more minutes and add more salt and pepper to taste.

12.   Turn the heat off and set aside for about minutes to let the ragout cool down a bit.

13.   Garnish with the optional parsley before serving and enjoy while warm or store.

Nutrition:

Calories: 77 kcal.

Carbs: 4.2g.

Fat: 4.1g.

Protein: 2.5g.

Fiber: 1.6g.

Sugar: 2.2g.

Pumpkin Pilaf

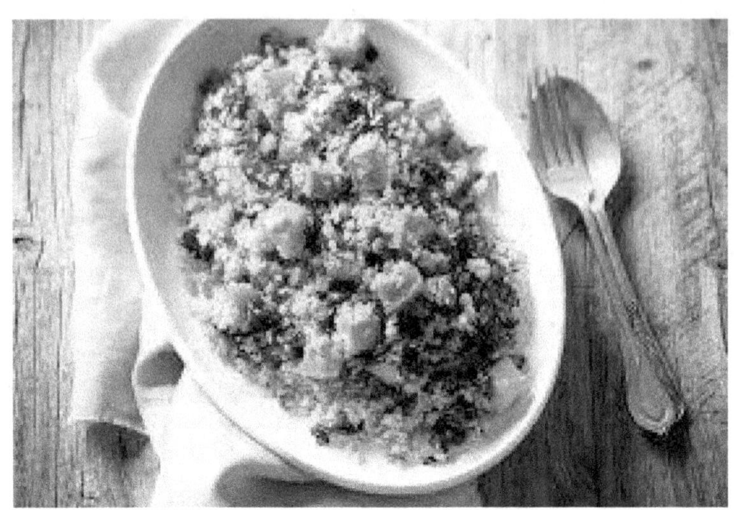

Serves: 2

Preparation Time: 20 minutes

Ingredients :

- 2 cup dry brown rice
- 2 tbsp. olive oil
- 1 sweet potato (medium, cubed)
- 2 cups fresh pumpkin (cubed)
- 2 cups kale (fresh or frozen)
- 2 celery ribs (medium, cut)
- 1 onion (medium, cut)
- 2 garlic cloves
- 1 tbsp. onion powder

- 1 bay leaf (chopped)
- Salt and black pepper to taste
- ½ cup pumpkin seeds (optional)
- Handful of fresh parsley (chopped, optional)

Directions:

1. Cook the rice according to the recipe.
2. Put a large skillet on medium heat and add the olive oil to the skillet.
3. Throw in the sweet potato and pumpkin cubes.
4. Add the kale, onion, celery, garlic and onion powder.
5. Cook the mixture for 15-20 minutes and turn the heat down to low.
6. Add the cooked rice, optional pumpkin seeds, a handful of fresh parsley and stir thoroughly.
7. Softly cook the mixture for another 5 minutes.
8. Enjoy or store the pilaf for another day!

Nutrition:

Calories: 557 kcal.

Carbs: 90.1g.

Fat: 16,8g.

Protein: 11.5g.

Fiber: 12.5g.

Sugar: 13.1g.

Chapter 11: Dinner Recipes

Baked Root Veg with Chili

Preparation time: 20 minutes

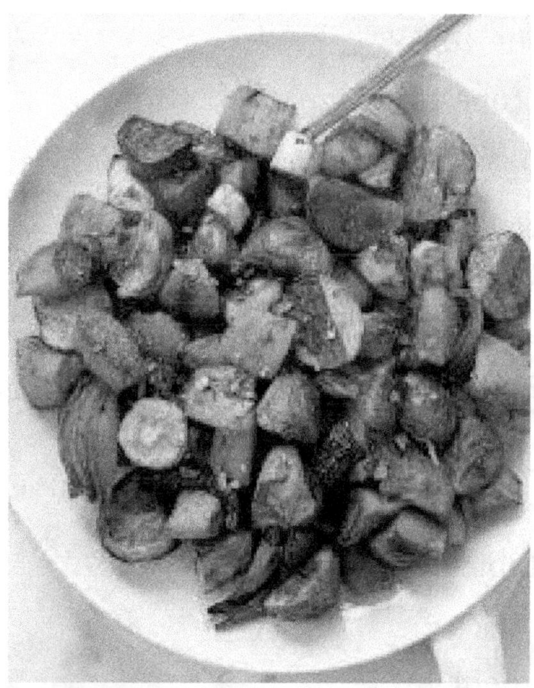

Serves: 2

Ingredients :

- Potatoes (three medium)

- Sweet potato (three medium)
- Yam (three small)
- Vegetable broth (two cups)
- Red kidney beans (one can)
- White kidney beans (one can)
- Diced tomatoes (two cans)
- Black beans (one can)
- Dried oregano (one teaspoon)
- Paprika (one and a half teaspoons)
- Cumin (two teaspoons)
- Chili powder (two tablespoons)
- Celery (two stalks)
- Carrots (two medium)
- Bell pepper (one large red)
- Red onion (two medium)
- Olive oil (two tablespoons)
- Cilantro (one bunch)
- Avocado (two medium)
- Bay leaf (one leaf)
- Sweet corn (one can)
- Tomato (two medium)
- Lime juice (two medium)

- Romaine (one head)

Directions:

1. Scrub and fork the potatoes and yams. Drizzle them with oil and quickly run over with clean hands. Sprinkle with salt and put on a baking tray for forty-five minutes or until you can pierce easily with a knife.

2. Heat the oil in a frying pan on medium and add the diced onion with the chopped bell pepper, diced carrots, and celery along with a quarter teaspoon of salt. Cook until the carrot is tender then add the paprika, oregano, cumin, and chili powder, along with the finely diced garlic.

3. Put in the full contents of the tomato cans, the bay leaf, and the vegetable broth.

4. Rinse all the cans of beans and drain well before adding to the pot. Stir the pot well and leave to simmer for a further thirty minutes. After this time has passed, get a potato masher and mash the chili to squish some of the beans and thicken the mixture.

5. At this point, you can add the juice of one lime, and salt and pepper to taste.

6. In separate bowls, prepare the fresh ingredients: finely dice the avocado and lightly mash with salt, pepper and the juice of another lime. Drain and rinse the corn and toss with half of the cilantro, finely chopped. Shred the romaine lettuce and dice the tomatoes.

7. Check that the root vegetables are done, remove from oven and slice open to cool slightly. Place in a nice dish and put on the table with a bowl of chili and all the sides for people to build their own masterpiece. You may also want to get vegan sour cream for this meal from the store. Enjoy!

Nutrition: calories: 63; protein: 4g; total fat: 14g; saturated fat: 2g; carbohydrates: 36g; fiber: 10g

Autumn Stuffed Enchiladas

Preparation time: 20 minutes

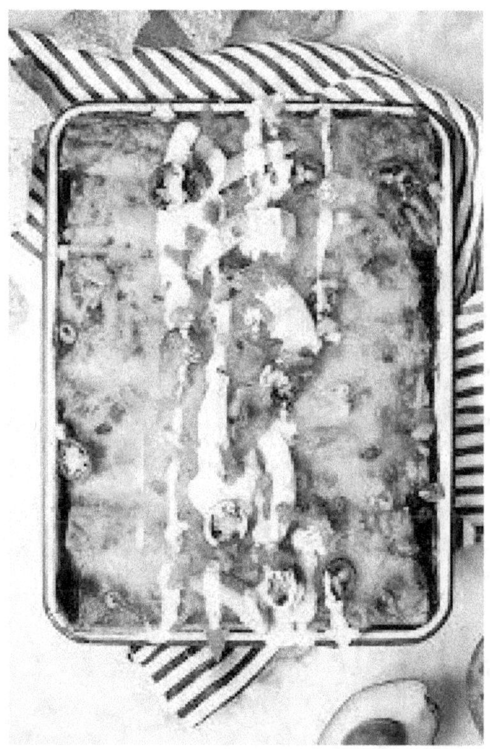

Serves: 2

Ingredients :

- Salt and pepper (to taste)
- Lemon juice (one medium lemon)
- Cashews (one cup raw)
- Cilantro (one bunch)
- Roasted pumpkin seeds (quarter cup)

- Corn tortillas (twelve pack)
- Butternut squash (two cups)
- Salsa (one and a half cups homemade or store-bought)
- Black beans (one can)
- Olive oil (two tablespoons)
- Cayenne pepper (quarter teaspoon)
- Chili flakes (one teaspoon)
- Cumin (one teaspoon)
- Garlic (three cloves)
- Jalapeno (one medium)
- Red onion (one small)
- Brussel sprouts (one cup)

Direction :

1. Soak the cashews in boiled water to cover and set aside.
2. Cut the squash in half and after scooping out the seeds, lightly rub olive oil with clean hands over the exposed flesh. Sprinkle with a little salt and pepper before putting on a baking sheet face

down. Cook for about forty-five minutes at 400F until it is cooked through.

3. Heat one tablespoon of olive oil in a frypan on medium heat and put chopped onion in, stirring until soft. Finely dice the jalapeno and garlic and finely slice the Brussel sprouts. Add these three things to the frypan and cook until the Brussels begin to wilt through.

4. Strain and rinse the black beans then add those to the frypan and mix well.

5. When the squash is cooked through and cool enough to handle, scrape out the soft insides away from the skin and put in a big bowl along with the Brussels mixture. Mix well again with the addition of generous pinches of salt and pepper to taste)

6. Put the tortillas in the oven to soften up (don't let them get crispy) while you get a baking dish out and very lightly oil the base and sides before spooning some salsa into it and doing the same. Spoon the squash mixture into the middle of the soft tortillas. Carefully roll them up to make little

open-ended wraps, then put in the baking dish with the open ends down to stop them from unrolling.

7. Do this for all twelve tortillas then pour the rest of the salsa on top and spread to evenly coat. Change the temperature of the oven to 350F and bake for thirty minutes.

8. While these cooks put the drained, soaked cashews into a blender with one and a half cups cold water, lemon juice, and a quarter teaspoon salt. Blend until smooth, adding tiny drizzles of water if it becomes too thick. This is your sour cream.

9. When enchiladas are done, leave to cool while you chop cilantro. Then drizzle the sour cream generously over the dish and top with cilantro and pumpkin seeds. Enjoy!

Nutrition: calories: 123; protein: 4g; total fat: 11g; saturated fat: 2g; carbohydrates: 36g; fiber: 10g

Creamy Vegetable Casserole

Preparation time: 20 minutes

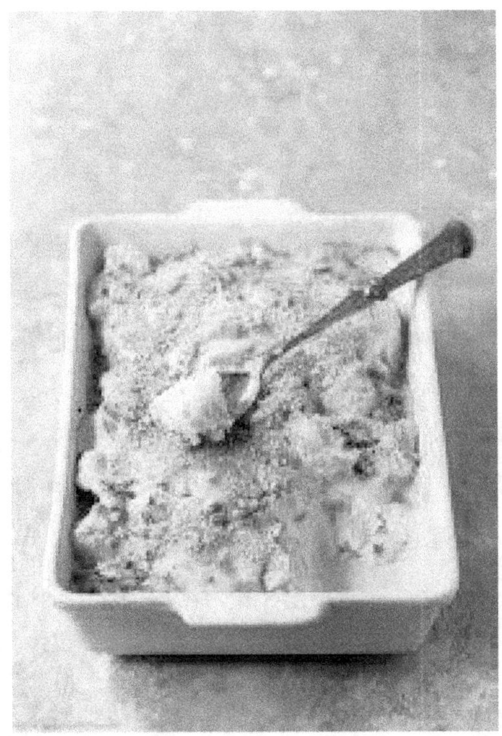

Serves: 2

Ingredients :

- Fresh rosemary (two tablespoons)
- Dried basil (one teaspoon)
- Dried oregano (one teaspoon)
- Garlic (three cloves)

- Nutritional yeast (half cup)
- Salt and pepper (to taste)
- Olive oil (two tablespoons)
- Apple cider vinegar (two tablespoons)
- Raw cashews (one cup)
- Zucchini (two large)
- Broccoli (one medium head)
- Cauliflower (one and a half medium head)
- Russet potatoes (ten medium)

Directions:

1. Pour boiled water over the cashews and leave to soak.
2. Cut up the cauliflower into small florets and boil until soft.
3. The potatoes in this dish will be similar to scalloped potatoes so they need to be sliced thinly. Cut carefully, but don't be too precise, just so long as they are as thin as you can get them (think really fat potato chips).
4. When the cauliflower is done, drain it and put it in a blender along with the drained cashews and one

and a half cups of cold water. Add a good half teaspoon of salt along with the apple cider vinegar and nutritional yeast. Blend until creamy.

5. Wash and grate the zucchini, set aside. Cut the broccoli into small bite-sized pieces and set aside.

6. In a large baking dish, spread the sides and bottom with generous amounts of olive oil. Then put two layers of potatoes down so that there are no gaps to the bottom.

7. Pour half of the cauliflower sauce to cover and spread evenly. Add the grated zucchini and spread out to cover the sauce. Sprinkle the oregano and basil over the zucchini, then push the pieces of broccoli into the zucchini to keep the surface as even as possible.

8. Drizzle a little more cauliflower sauce around the broccoli pieces to fill in the gaps. Do another layer to use up the rest of the potatoes, then pour the rest of the sauce over top of that. Spread it out as evenly as possible, right to the edges to fill in all the gaps around the sides.

9. Sprinkle the top with a half teaspoon of black pepper and a generous pinch or two of salt. Finely chop the fresh rosemary and sprinkle that on top also. Put in the oven on 400F for forty-five minutes. It will be done when a knife pierces the potatoes without pulling them up and the top should be beautifully browned. Let it cool before serving and enjoy!

10. Pasta – Italian, cheesy, decadent, lasagnas; all the words that mean love and care and satisfaction. These recipes will help you share the love with your guests and remind you what true self-love is when you make them for yourself. Indulgence doesn't have to be unhealthy.

Nutrition: calories: 89; protein: 6g; total fat: 4g; saturated fat: 1g; carbohydrates: 37g; fiber: 10g

Butternut Squash Alfredo

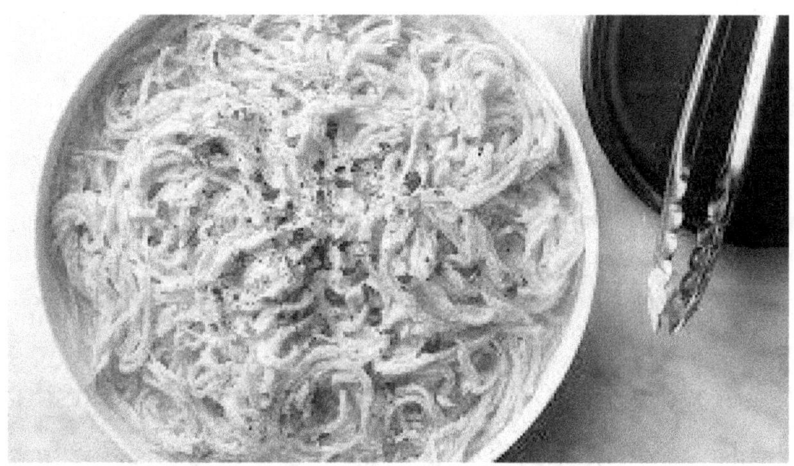

Ingredients :

- Whole grain linguine (three cups)

- Vegetable broth (two cups)

- Butternut Squash (three cups diced)

- Salt (quarter teaspoon)

- Paprika (one teaspoon)

- Black pepper (half teaspoon)

- Garlic (two cloves)

- White onion (one medium)

- Green peas (one cup)

- Zucchini (one large)

- Olive oil (two tablespoons)

- Sage (two tablespoons fresh)

Directions:

1. Heat the oil in a large frypan with medium heat. While it heats, ensures the sage leaves are clean and dry, then put in the oil to fry, moving around to not burn. Pull them out and put them on a paper towel.
2. Into the frypan, put the peeled and diced squash along with paprika, diced onion, and black pepper. Cook until the onion is soft then add the broth and salt to taste. Bring to a boil before turning down to low heat and leaving the squash to cook through.
3. In another pot, cook the linguine in water with a little salt.
4. When the squash is tender, put it in a blender along with all the liquid and other ingredients. Blend until creamy and taste to see if more salt, pepper or spice is needed. Put it back in the frypan to keep warm on low heat.

5. Using a grater, grate the zucchini lengthwise to make long noodles. Make as many long ones as you can to blend in with the linguine. Add them to the sauce along with the green peas and cook in the butternut squash for five minutes.

6. When the pasta is done, save one cup of liquid before you drain it. Add the linguine to the pasta and stir well to coat the linguine. If the sauce is too thick, add a little of the reserved pasta water.

7. Serve the pasta topped with the fried sage leaves and a little more black pepper. Enjoy!

Nutrition: calories: 32; protein: 4g; total fat: 14g; saturated fat: 2g; carbohydrates: 36g; fiber: 10g

Vegan Lasagna

Preparation time: 20 minutes

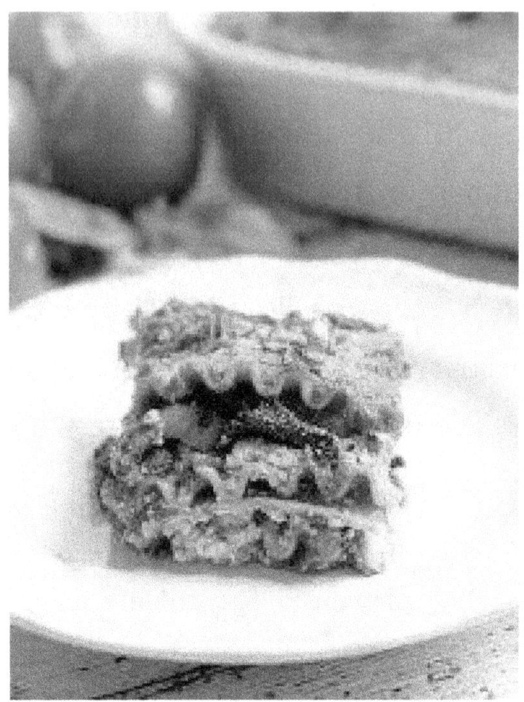

S erves: 2

Ingredients :

- Tapioca starch (four tablespoons)
- Salt (half teaspoon)
- Apple cider vinegar (one tablespoon)
- Lemon juice (four medium lemons)
- Raw cashews (one and a half cups)
- Baby spinach (three cups)

- Lasagna noodles (one box)

- Zucchini (two medium)

- Garlic powder (half teaspoon)

- Dried oregano (two teaspoons)

- Dried basil (two teaspoons)

- Salt (one teaspoon)

- Olive oil (two tablespoons)

- Nutritional yeast (half cup)

- Firm tofu (one pack)

- Tomato puree (one mini can)

- Onion powder (one tablespoon)

- Garlic (six bulbs)

- White onion (one medium)

- Salt and pepper (to taste)

- Crushed tomatoes (two cans)

- Dried red lentils (one cup dried)

Directions:

1. Put three cups of water in a saucepan with the lentils, then bring to a boil before reducing to a simmer for around twenty minutes. Drain the lentils and set aside.

2. In the same saucepan, add oil and the diced onion and let cook down. When the onion is soft, add finely diced garlic, generous pinches of salt and pepper, one teaspoon each of dried oregano and basil, the two cans of crushed tomato and the one can of tomato puree. Leave to simmer for fifteen minutes, stirring every five minutes. Add the lentils to this then set aside, this is the chunky marinara.

3. Put half a cup of cashews into a bowl with two cups of boiled water and set aside.

4. Wash and slice the zucchini into lengthwise strips that are long and relatively thin then set aside.

5. Put one cup of cashews in a blender and pulse until crumbly. Break up the tofu and add to the blender along with the juice from one lemon, one teaspoon each of basil and oregano, the nutritional yeast, garlic powder, and a little salt. Keep pulsing until it is mostly smooth but still a little textured. Put into a bowl and set aside, this is your ricotta.

6. Drain the soaked cashews and put them into a clean blender with the apple cider vinegar, the juice from one lemon, tapioca starch, and a little salt. Pour in one and a half cups of water and blend until smooth. Pour this into a saucepan on medium heat and stir until it becomes stretchy then set aside. This is the cheese sauce.

7. In a large baking dish, place a few spoonfuls of the marinara sauce and spread it to cover the bottom and sides of the dish. Begin to layer the lasagna noodles, the ricotta, the zucchini, and the cheese sauce. Follow this with half of the spinach, more marinara, lasagna noodles, ricotta, spinach, and the cheese sauce. Keep repeating until all ingredients have been used except for a small portion of the cheese sauce.

8. Put into a 350F oven for one hour on the highest shelf. Remove after forty minutes and spoon the remainder of the cheese sauce over the top to resemble mozzarella blobs, then return to the oven for twenty more minutes. Let rest then serve and enjoy!

Nutrition: calories: 43; protein: 4g; total fat: 14g; saturated fat: 2g; carbohydrates: 36g; fiber: 10g

Creamy, Dreamy Dahl

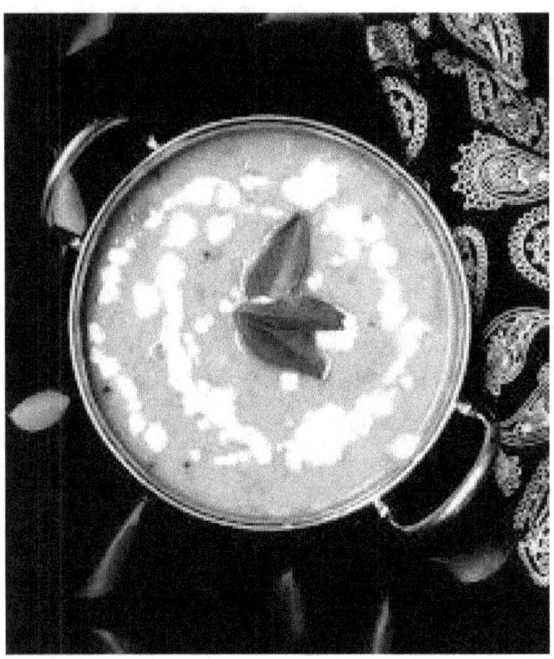

Preparation time: 20 minutes

Serves: 2

Ingredients :

- Fresh cilantro (small bunch)

- Lemon juice (half one medium)

- Red lentils (one cup dried)

- Tomato (one medium)

- Salt (three-quarter teaspoon)

- Paprika (half teaspoon)

- Ground cardamom (half teaspoon)

- Turmeric (half teaspoon)

- Fresh ginger (one tablespoon minced)

- Garlic (four cloves)

- Jalapeno (one medium)

- White onion (two medium)

- Cinnamon (one stick or quarter teaspoon ground)

- Cumin (half teaspoon)

- Coconut oil (two tablespoons)

- Coconut milk (half can)

- Basmati rice (one cup)

Directions:

1. Rinse the lentils then put in a saucepan with three cups of water and cook for twenty minutes on medium heat.

2. Chop the onion and finely dice the ginger, jalapeno, and garlic. Dice the tomatoes too and set aside.

3. Heat one tablespoon oil in a frypan on medium and put the cumin and cinnamon in the oil to release the aromas for one minute, then add the onions. Let them sweat a little before adding the garlic, ginger, and jalapeno.

4. In another saucepan, fill with rinsed rice, then top with water to cover. Add one tablespoon of coconut oil and the coconut milk (the liquid should be one inch above rice) and give it a quick stir. Cook on medium-high until it boils, then put the lid on and turn the heat down to medium-low and leave to simmer.

5. After a few minutes, put the salt, paprika, cardamom, and turmeric into the mix along with the diced tomato. If you used a cinnamon stick, pull it out now. Leave this on low to cook through.

6. When the lentils are done, drain them and put them back on the stove top. Scrape the tomato

mixture into the lentils, along with the lemon juice and salt if needed. Mix well.

7. Check on the rice, and if the water has been absorbed and the rice can be easily fluffed up with a fork then it should be ready. Chop cilantro and top each serving of rice and dahl. Enjoy!

Nutrition: calories: 166; protein: 4g; total fat: 14g; saturated fat: 2g; carbohydrates: 36g; fiber: 10g

Easy Thai Coconut Curry

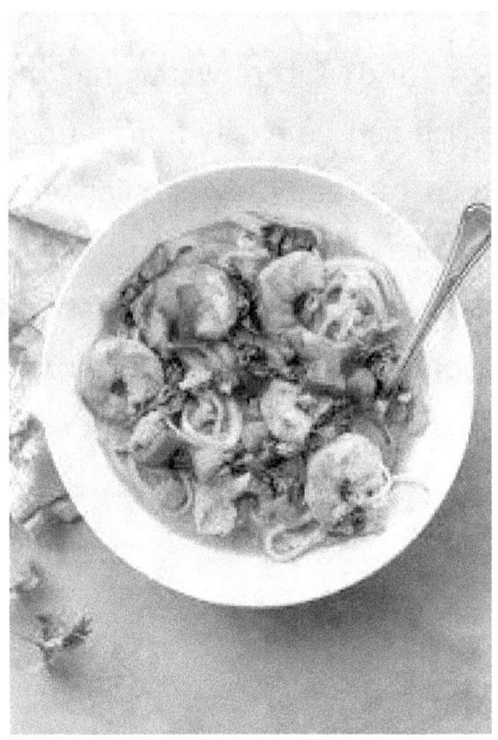

Preparation time: 20 minutes

Serves: 2

Ingredients :

- Jasmine rice (one cup)
- Fresh basil leaves (quarter cup)
- Kaffir lime leaves (three leaves)
- Whole peppercorns (two tablespoons)

- Snap peas (one cup)

- Eggplant (one small)

- Fresh ginger (one teaspoon grated)

- Garlic (three cloves)

- Lime juice (one medium lime)

- Coconut oil (four tablespoons)

- Maple syrup (one teaspoon)

- Soy sauce (one tablespoon)

- Firm tofu (one package)

- Thai red curry paste (three tablespoons)

- Coconut milk (one can)

Directions:

1. In a bowl, mix half the can of coconut milk with the soy sauce, maple syrup and curry paste.

2. Drain the tofu and cut into small cubes. Finely dice two cloves of garlic, grate the ginger and set aside. Cut the eggplant into small pieces, toss them in generous amounts of salt and set aside in a bowl.

3. In another saucepan, put one tablespoon coconut oil and heat on medium. Dice the last clove of

garlic and put into the oil along with the rice. Stir around as the garlic cooks and the oil coats the rice. When some of the rice starts to get a little toasted, pour in water to just cover the rice and add the other half can of coconut milk along with one kefir lime leaf. Wait for it to come to a boil, then put the lid on, change heat to low and let it simmer without touching it.

4. Heat one tablespoon oil in a large frypan on medium and put in the tofu, cooking until all sides have been fried and are browned. Set the tofu aside.

5. Put in two more tablespoons of oil and put in the ginger and garlic and let fry for one minute. Rinse the salt off the eggplant, drain and put the eggplant in with the ginger and garlic.

6. When the eggplant gets a little soft and a little color, then add the snap peas and change heat to high. Put the curry mix into the pan and also the tofu and two of the lime leaves along with the peppercorns.

7. Cook for another two minutes while stirring to get everything coated and combined.

8. Check on the rice, it will be done when there is no liquid left and the rice can be fluffed easily with a fork. Remove the lime leaf and spoon rice onto plates.

9. Slice up the basil and quickly stir through the curry before spooning it over the rice. Finish with a generous squeeze of lime over everything and enjoy!

Nutrition: calories: 60; protein: 4g; total fat: 14g; saturated fat: 2g; carbohydrates: 36g; fiber: 10g

Sabrosa Spanish Paella

Preparation time: 20 minutes

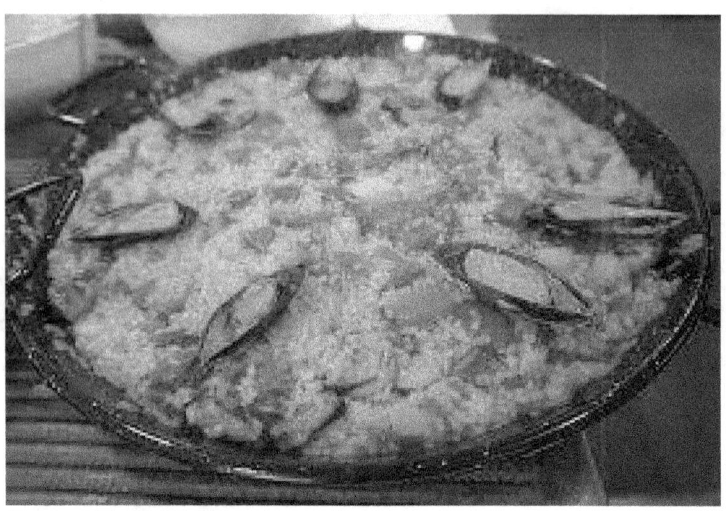

Serves: 2

Ingredients :

- Paprika (one teaspoon)
- Cayenne (half teaspoon)
- Saffron (one pinch)
- Capers (two tablespoons)
- Garlic (two cloves)
- Red bell pepper (three medium)
- Artichoke hearts (two small jars)
- Portobello mushrooms (three cups)
- Lime (one medium)

- White onion (one medium)

- Salt and pepper (to taste)

- Olive oil (three tablespoons)

- Nutritional yeast (two tablespoons)

- Saffron rice (two cups)

- White wine (two cups)

- Vegetable stock (six cups)

Directions:

1. Heat a large soup pot on medium-high and put in four cups of the vegetable stock and all of the wine. Let it boil before adding all the rice, then put the lid on and allow to simmer for fifteen minutes.

2. Turn on the oven at 375F.

3. Put two red bell peppers on a baking tray and cut them in half then rub with olive oil using clean hands so they are well coated. Put in the oven cut side down and cook for twenty minutes or until they get all wrinkly and start to look a little burnt.

4. Get an oven-safe large frypan (if you don't have one, then use a regular frypan and get an oven

dish ready for later) and heat a tablespoon of olive oil on medium before adding diced onions and one thinly sliced bell pepper.

5. After the onions and bell pepper become soft, put in the sliced mushrooms and leave for five more minutes.

6. Put into the frypan the cayenne, paprika, and saffron and stir around. Then put in the finely diced garlic, capers and artichoke hearts (without the liquid).

7. When the bell peppers are ready from the oven, let them cool before pulling off their skins then chop them into small slices and add to the frypan.

8. Drain the rice and then put in the frypan and mix well. Add generous amounts of salt and pepper at this point and taste.

9. If you used an oven-safe frypan, then put it into the oven. If you didn't, then transfer the pan contents into an oven dish and put that in instead.

10.   After ten minutes, pull out the dish and add one cup of vegetable broth and mix through really

well. Do this again after another ten minutes, then remove ten minutes later. The paella should have been in the oven for a total of thirty minutes.

11.   Cut up a lime into wedges and scatter about the dish. Roughly chop fresh parsley and scatter this over top also along with the nutritional yeast. Enjoy!

12.   ROASTS – Going vegan doesn't mean you have to give up the traditional roast, if anything, it means you get to experience unique flavors and textures that you never knew existed!

Nutrition: calories: 234; protein: 4g; total fat: 14g; saturated fat: 2g; carbohydrates: 36g; fiber: 10g

Vegan Festive Nut Roast

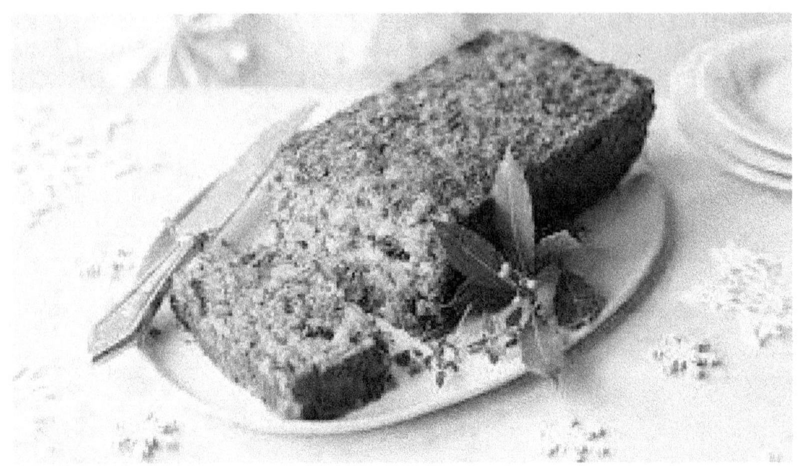

Preparation time: 20 minutes

Serves: 2

Ingredients:

- Paprika (two teaspoons)
- Tomato puree (one teaspoon)
- Miso paste (two teaspoons)
- Dried rosemary (half teaspoon)
- Dried sage (half teaspoon)
- Dried thyme (half teaspoon)
- Tahini (one tablespoon)
- Dried breadcrumbs (one cup)

- Chestnuts (one small can)
- Raw cashews (one cup)
- Carrots (one and a half cups)
- Fresh rosemary (two sprigs)
- Fresh thyme (two sprigs)
- Butternut squash (one and a half cups)
- Olive oil (one tablespoon)
- Garlic (two cloves)
- Onion (one medium)

Directions:

1. Peel and chop carrots and squash into small pieces then boil until they are very tender.
2. Put cashews and chestnuts into a blender and pulse until they are ground but not too fine.
3. Heat oil in a frypan over medium and put in chopped onion until softens. Finely dice garlic and put that in too.
4. Mash the carrots and squash in a bowl then add the onions and nuts. Mix very well then add every other ingredient. Well-oil a loaf sized dish and pack in firmly.

5. Bake at 350F covered with foil for one hour, then take off the foil and bake for another fifteen minutes.
6. Flip it out onto a plate and top with fresh thyme and rosemary, serve with cranberry sauce and mushroom gravy.

Nutrition: calories: 542; protein: 4g; total fat: 14g; saturated fat: 2g; carbohydrates: 36g; fiber: 10g

Roasted Vegetable Pie

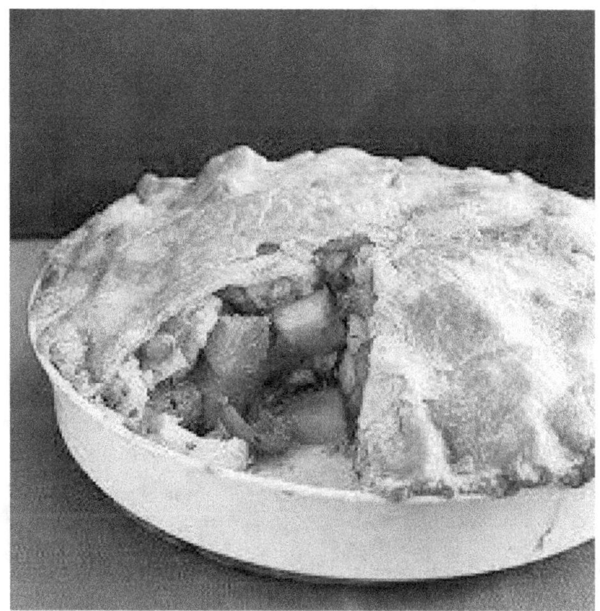

Preparation time: 20 minutes

Serves: 2

Ingredients :

- Vegetable suet or vegetable shortening (one cup)
- White flour (one and two-thirds cup)
- Salt and pepper (to taste)
- Cranberry sauce (one tablespoon)
- English mustard (one teaspoon)
- Fresh thyme (two teaspoons)

- Hazelnuts (one-third cup)
- Chestnuts (one small can)
- Butter beans (one can)
- Dried cranberries (quarter cup)
- Mushrooms (three cups)
- Garlic (two cloves)
- Olive oil (one tablespoon)
- Leeks (one cup)
- Onions (two medium)

Directions:

1. Heat oil in a frypan and put in the finely sliced leeks and onions. Let cook down for five minutes before adding the finely diced garlic. Put in the cranberries, drained and rinsed beans and chestnuts, chopped hazelnuts, sliced mushrooms, mustard, and thyme. Add generous pinches of salt and pepper then stir for ten minutes.

2. Sift flour and a half teaspoon of salt into a bowl and make a well in the middle.

3. Put two-thirds of a cup of water in a saucepan and bring to the boil then stir in the suet to melt.

4. Pour into the well of flour and gently fold the flour in until combined enough to knead. Do so for five minutes then set aside.

5. Oil a springform cake tin then roll out three-quarters of the pastry to lay into the tin. Spoon the cranberry sauce onto the base to cover then spoon in the vegetables.

6. Roll out the last quarter of the pastry and cover the vegetables. Run a knife around the edge of the lip to take off the extra pastry, then press down around the edges with a fork to pinch closed the top and base.

7. Drizzle and rub a tiny bit of oil over the top of the pie before you put it in the oven for one hour.

8. Let it sit for ten minutes before carefully lifting the sides of the cake tin and sliding the pie off the base onto a plate. Enjoy!

Nutrition: calories: 188; protein: 4g; total fat: 14g; saturated fat: 2g; carbohydrates: 36g; fiber: 10g

Epic Vegan Holiday Roast

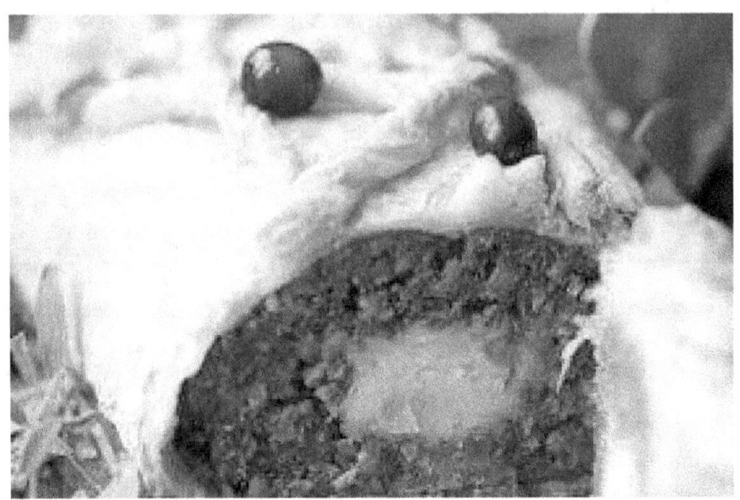

Preparation time: 20 minutes

Serves: 2

Ingredients :

- Salt and pepper (to taste)
- Ground sage (three teaspoons)
- Onion powder (three-quarter teaspoon)
- Garlic powder (one teaspoon)
- Soy sauce (one teaspoon)
- Maple syrup (one teaspoon)
- Miso paste (one tablespoon)
- Olive oil (three tablespoons)

- Pinto beans (half a can)
- Vegetable broth (four cups)
- Vital wheat gluten (two and quarter cups)
- Sourdough bread (one small uncut round loaf)
- Fresh parsley (half cup)
- Fresh thyme (four sprigs)
- Dried rosemary (one teaspoon)
- Dried thyme (one tablespoon)
- Mushrooms (four cups)
- Garlic (five cloves)
- Celery (one cup)
- White onion (one large)
- Barbeque sauce (two tablespoons)
- Teriyaki sauce (two tablespoons)

Directions:

1. For the stuffing, dice the sourdough loaf into bite-sized chunks and spread over a baking tray. Bake for fifteen minutes at 350F tossing every five minutes.

2. Heat two tablespoons oil in a large frypan on medium and put diced onion and celery into it.

When soft, add four cloves of diced garlic followed by diced mushrooms and another tablespoon of oil. Put in chopped fresh parsley with the dried rosemary, one tablespoon dried sage and the dried thyme.

3. When the mushrooms have cooked down, put in two cups of vegetable broth and generous sprinkles of salt and pepper. After it has simmered for five minutes, use a slotted spoon to pull out all the vegetables and put into a bowl with the bread chunks. Mix through really well then using a regular spoon, add the remaining liquid to the bread mixture until the bread has absorbed as much as it can without feeling soggy.

4. Oil a large baking dish and spread the contents into it before covering with aluminum wrap. Turn oven up to 375F and bake for thirty minutes covered and another twenty minutes uncovered. Set aside then turn the oven up again to 400F

5. In a blender put one teaspoon of sage with the onion and garlic powders. Put in one tablespoon of olive oil with the maple syrup, miso paste and

one clove of whole garlic. Rinse the beans and put in along with one and a half cups of vegetable broth and one teaspoon of salt. Blend well until smooth and put into a big bowl then put in the vital wheat gluten and mix until it becomes dough-like. Use clean hands to work it (think of it like making bread) until it feels stretchy and uniforms then knead for another two minutes.

6. Use a rolling pin to roll it out to the size of your baking dish in a rectangle shape.

7. Spoon the stuffing down the center of the dough lengthwise. It should be stuffed so that when you roll it over, you have just enough dough left to pinch it together around the stuffing center. Do this the whole way down until you have a log. The stuffing should be densely packed inside so pack more in from each end if there's room.

8. Roll in oiled aluminum foil tightly and twist each end like a giant wrapped candy so that the roast is very tight. Put into a baking dish and pour the last half cup of broth around it like a bath and bake for ninety minutes but make sure you turn it

every twenty minutes so that all sides get a chance on the bottom.

9. You know it's done when it feels firm to the touch much like a cooked meatloaf. Carefully unwrap the foil and put it back into the baking dish with a little drizzle of oil to stop it sticking.

10. Whisk together the BBQ and teriyaki sauces and pour over the roast making sure it is all coated. Put the fresh thyme sprigs on top and cook for a further ten minutes until the glaze gets sticky and darkens.

11. Let it rest for ten minutes then cut into rings and serve with mushroom gravy and cranberry sauce.

Nutrition: calories: 238; protein: 4g; total fat: 14g; saturated fat: 2g; carbohydrates: 36g; fiber: 10g

Chapter 12: Desserts Recipes

Healthy Salted Caramel Bar

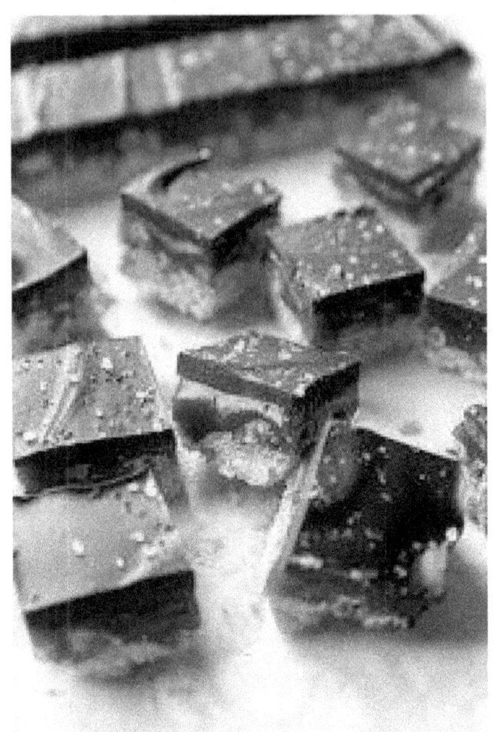

Preparation time: 30 minutes

Serves: 2

Ingredients :

- Almond milk (two tablespoons)
- Maple syrup (two tablespoons)
- Vanilla extract (one and quarter teaspoons)
- Cocoa powder (third cup)

- Coconut oil (half cup)
- Salt (quarter teaspoon)
- Cashew butter (quarter cup)
- Almond milk (two teaspoons)
- Medjool dates (one and a half cup)
- Shredded coconut (half cup)
- Almond flour (one cup)

Directions:

1. In a food processor put coconut oil, four dates, shredded coconut, and almond flour and blend. Evenly push it into a baking paper lined slice pan and put it in the freezer.
2. Next, using the processor again, put the rest of the dates along with the salt, one teaspoon vanilla, almond milk, and cashew butter. Blend until smooth and add to the top of the slice pan and put back in the freezer.
3. Heat the coconut oil in a saucepan on low and mix in the cocoa powder, quarter teaspoon vanilla with the maple syrup and stir until a consistent texture.

4. Pour this over the slice pan once it has cooled off, top with a sprinkling of shredded coconut, and put it in the fridge for two hours. Slice and enjoy!

Nutrition: calories 76, fat 1, fiber 9, carbs 6, protein 5

Chocolate Avocado Pudding

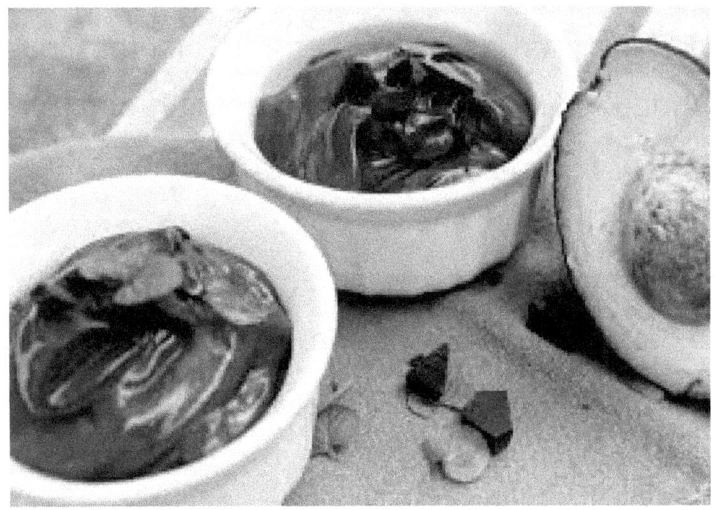

Preparation time: 30 minutes

Serves: 2

Ingredients :

- Maple syrup (quarter cup)

- Salt (pinch)
- Vanilla extract (half teaspoon)
- Almond milk (four tablespoons)
- Cocoa powder (quarter cup)
- Vegan dark chocolate chips (quarter cup)
- Ripe avocados (two medium)

Directions:

1. Heat a saucepan over medium and bring to a simmer the maple syrup and the almond milk. Take off the heat and stir in the chocolate chips to melt then set aside to cool.
2. Put everything else in a food processor then add in the milk mixture and blend until 100% smooth.
3. Spoon into individual portion containers, cover and put in the fridge until set. Enjoy!

Nutrition: calories 65, fat 1, fiber 2, carbs 4, protein 5

Decadent Chocolate Cake

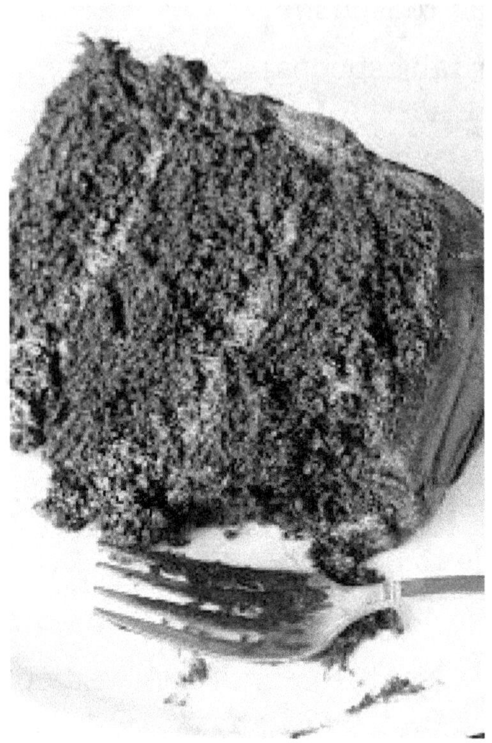

Preparation time: 30 minutes

Serves: 2

Ingredients :

- Vanilla extract (two teaspoons)
- Almond butter (two tablespoons)
- Almond milk (two and quarter cups)
- Icing sugar (two and a half cups)

- Cocoa powder (one and quarter cups)
- Dark chocolate vegan chips (quarter cups)
- Apple cider vinegar (two teaspoons)
- Vegan butter (three-quarter cup)
- Applesauce (one cup)
- Coconut oil (half cup)
- Salt (quarter cup)
- Baking powder (half teaspoon)
- Baking soda (three teaspoons)
- Raw cane sugar (one and a half cups)
- Flour (two and a half cups)

Directions:

1. Get a large bowl and sift into it the flour, baking powder, baking soda, sugar, salt and a three-quarter cup of cocoa and stir through.
2. In a saucepan on low heat melt the coconut oil quickly then take off the heat. Put in the vinegar, one teaspoon vanilla, applesauce and two cups of the milk then mix well.
3. Put everything together and mix with an electric beater until it's really smooth.

4. Pour into two 8-inch cake pans lined with baking paper and bake for forty-five minutes at 350F. Check by inserting a knife to the center at an angle, if the knife is clean when you remove it, then it is cooked through. Leave to cool.

5. In a clean saucepan, melt together the vegan butter and chocolate chips on low heat while stirring.

6. In a bowl, sift in the rest of the cocoa powder with the icing sugar, one teaspoon vanilla, almond butter and the rest of the almond milk. Pour in the chocolate butter and mix with an electric beater until thick and creamy.

7. Slice the very top off of one cake to make it flat and spoon some frosting on top. Spread it around before adding the second cake. Ice the entire double-stacked cake with the rest of the icing, starting with the top and then moving the icing down around the edges.

8. Sprinkle the top with whatever you like! Chocolate shavings or shredded coconut, chopped nuts or berries. Enjoy!

Nutrition: calories 54, fat 1, fiber 2, carbs 6, protein 5

Vegan Cheesecake with Blueberries

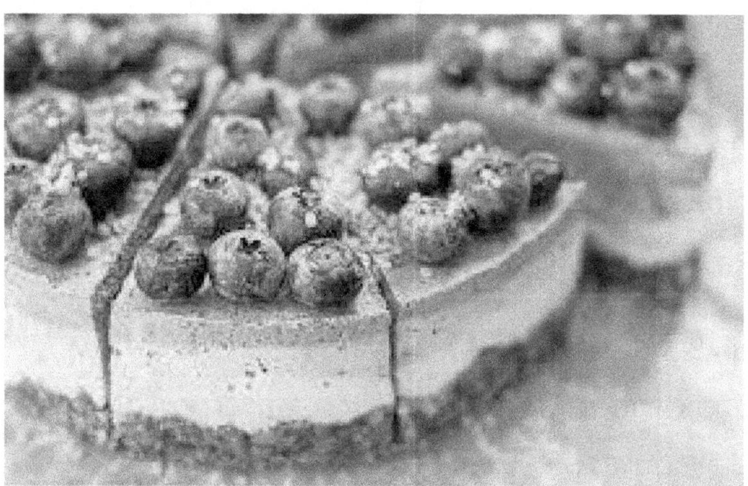

Preparation time: 30 minutes

Serves: 2

Ingredients :

- Chia seeds (one tablespoon)
- Lemon juice (three tablespoons)
- Blueberries (one cup fresh or frozen)
- Freeze-dried blueberries (quarter cup)

- Vanilla extract (one tablespoon)
- Maple syrup (third cup)
- Coconut oil (quarter cup plus two tablespoons)
- Coconut milk (half cup)
- Raw cashews (two cups)
- Salt (quarter teaspoon)
- Cinnamon (one teaspoon)
- Dates (two)
- Almond flour (half cup)
- Raw pecans (half cup)

Directions:

1. Soak the cashews in boiled water an hour before starting and set aside.
2. In a food processor, put the pecans along with the pitted dates, two tablespoons coconut oil, almond flour, salt, and cinnamon and blend to a slightly choppy, nutty dough.
3. Press into the base of a six-inch cake tin that is either a well-oiled springform tin or a baking paper lined regular cake tin that will enable the cheesecake to be lifted out when done.

4. In the same processor, put the soaked and drained cashews with the coconut milk, maple syrup, remaining coconut oil, two tablespoons of lemon juice and vanilla. Blend until creamy, adding a little more coconut milk if necessary. If the filling needs more of anything, now is the time to add it; either vanilla, lemon, salt or syrup.

5. Pour two thirds over the nut base and drop the pan on the counter a few times to let it settle before placing in the freezer.

6. Put the freeze-dried berries into the rest of the mixture and blend to a beautiful purple filling and pour over the top of the cheesecake, dropping as before to settle.

7. In a blender, put the chia seeds, a tablespoon of lemon and whole blueberries. Blend and pour over the top before putting back into the freezer for three hours.

8. Remove from the cake tin before serving and slice with a warm knife. Enjoy!

Nutrition: calories 76, fat 8, fiber 2, carbs 6, protein 5

Do the Cocoa Shake

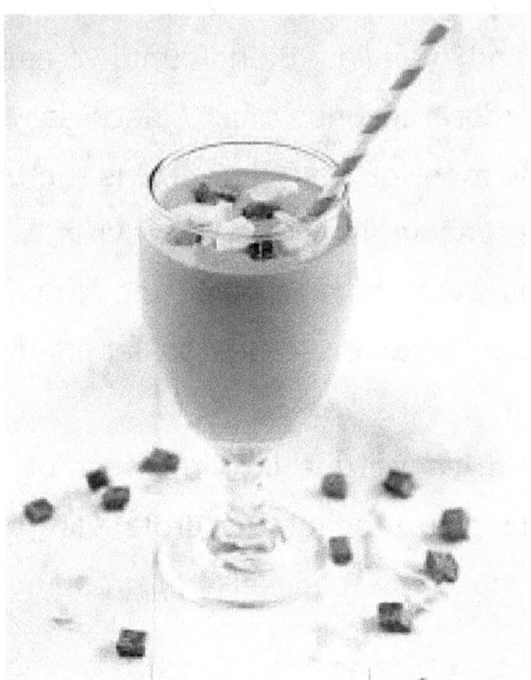

Servings: 4 servings, 1 cup (235 ml) per serving

Protein content per serving: **11 g**

Ingredients

- 12 ounces (340 g) soft silken tofu
- 1 (355 ml) unsweetened plain or vanilla vegan milk of choice

- ¼ cup (80 g) agave nectar or pure maple syrup, adjust to taste
- ¼ cup (64 g) natural creamy peanut or almond butter, slightly salted is fine
- ¼ cup (20 g) unsweetened cocoa powder
- 1 teaspoon pure vanilla extract
- 2 tablespoons (20 g) hemp powder, optional
- 1 frozen banana (peeled before freezing in a plastic sandwich bag), optional
- Ice cubes, optional

Direction

1. Combine all the ingredients in a blender and blend until perfectly smooth. Add hemp powder for an extra boost of protein, a sliced frozen banana for a thicker and fruitier shake, or ice cubes for a colder, thicker shake without any added flavor.

2. Serve immediately or refrigerate for later use: be sure to only add the ice cubes upon serving, if storing for later. Stir well or blend again if adding ice cubes.

Nutrition: calories 150, fat 1, fiber 9, carbs 6, protein 5

Smoky Bean and Tempeh Patties

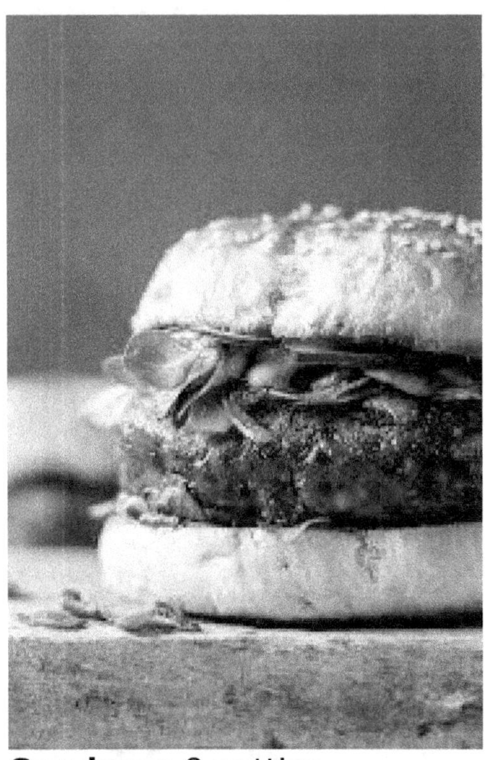

Servings: 8 patties

Protein content per patty: **10 g**

Ingredients

- 1 cup (177 g) cooked cannellini beans 8 ounces (227 g) tempeh
- '¼ cup (91 g) cooked bulgur
- 2 cloves garlic, pressed
- ¼ teaspoons onion powder
- 4 teaspoons (20 ml) liquid smoke
- 4 teaspoons (20 ml) vegan Worcestershire sauce
- 1 teaspoon smoked paprika
- 2 tablespoons (30 g) organic ketchup
- 2 tablespoons (40 g) pure maple syrup
- 2 tablespoons (30 ml) neutral-flavored oil
- 3 tablespoons (45 ml) tamari.'
- ¼ cup (60 g) chickpea flour
- Nonstick cooking spray

Direction

1. Mash the beans in a large bowl: It's okay if a few small pieces of beans are left. Crumble (do not mash) the tempeh into small pieces on top. Add the bulgur and garlic. In a medium bowl, whisk together the remaining ingredients, except the flour and cooking spray. Stir into the crumbled

tempeh preparation. Add the flour and mix until well combined. Chill for 1 hour before shaping into patties.

2. Preheat the oven to 350°F (180°C. or gas mark 4). Line a baking sheet with parchment paper. Scoop out a packed 1/3 cup (96 g) per patty, shaping into an approximately 3-inch (8 cm) circle and flattening slightly on the prepared sheet. You should get eight 3.5-inch (9 cm) patties in all. Lightly coat the top of the patties with cooking spray. Bake for 15 minutes, carefully flip, lightly coat the top of the patties with cooking spray, and bake for another 15 minutes until lightly browned and firm.

3. Leftovers can be stored in an airtight container in the refrigerator for up to 4 days. The patties can also be frozen, tightly wrapped in foil, for up to 3 months.

4. If you don't eat all the patties at once, reheat the leftovers on low heat in a skillet lightly greased with olive oil or cooking spray for about 5 minutes on each side until heated through.

Nutrition: calories 130, fat 1, fiber 2, carbs 6, protein 8

Spelt and Seed Rolls

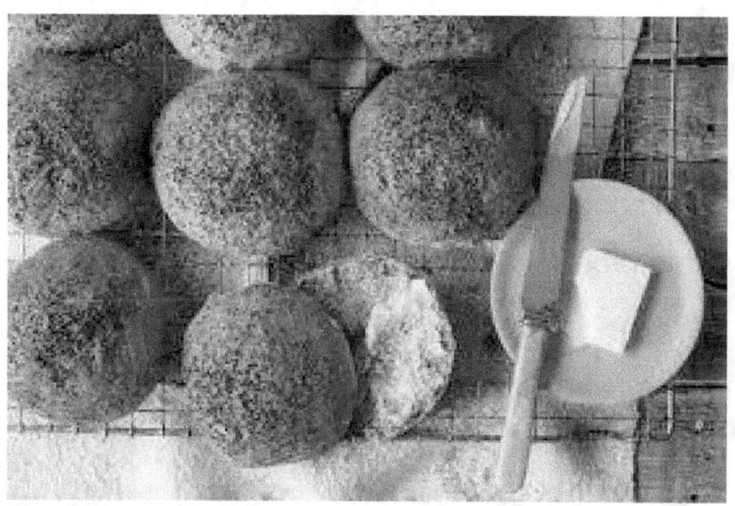

Servings: 9 rolls

Protein content per roll: **15 g**

Ingredients

- 1 cup (235 ml) unsweetened plain vegan milk, lukewarm
- 2 teaspoons apple cider vinegar
- ⅓ cup (120 ml) water, lukewarm

- 2 tablespoons (30 ml) neutral-flavored oil
- 2 tablespoons (40 g) agave nectar
- 3 cups plus scant
- ⅓ cup (480 g) whole spelt flour, divided
- ¼ cup (30 g) oat flour or finely ground oats
- ¼ cup (36 g) vital wheat gluten
- 3 tablespoons (30 g) shelled hemp seeds
- 3 tablespoons (25 g) sunflower seeds
- 2 tablespoons (15 g) golden roasted flaxseeds
- 2 tablespoons (24 g) chia seeds
- 1 tablespoon (7 g) caraway seeds or (9 g) poppy seeds
- 1 teaspoon fine sea salt
- 2 teaspoons instant yeast

Direction

1. Combine milk and vinegar in a measuring cup. Allow two minutes to milk. This is your "license."
2. Add water, oil and agave (or maple syrup or molasses) to the butter. Set aside.

3. In a bowl, place a 3A cup (450 g) of ground flour, oatmeal, wheat gluten, whole grains, salt, and yeast. Pour the wet ingredients over the dry ones.

4. Knead the dough with a stand mixer for 10 minutes until the dough becomes soft and not too dry or too sticky. If necessary, gently add 1 tablespoon (15 ml).

5. Cover for 75 minutes or until doubled.

6. Hit the dough. Place on a soft baking sheet, lightly smooth and form a circular disk approximately 10 inches (25 cm) long. Cover both sides of the disc with flour. Make 9 equal triangles from the center, similar to the buns. You can shape them or put them in round loaves.

7. Slowly sprinkle the extra flour and place it back on a baking sheet. Slowly lower by pressing the palm of your hand. Cover with plastic wrap. Let it grow for 25 minutes.

8. While the rolls rise, heat the oven to 400 degrees Fahrenheit (200 degrees Celsius, or gas mark 6). Remove the plastic wrap and do not brown or hollow it for 20 to 22 minutes or until it touches

the bottom of the roll. Let cool on a rack. Store the rest in an airtight container at room temperature. Roulette is best enjoyed fresh, but it will last up to 2 days.

Nutrition: calories 56, fat 1, fiber 2, carbs 4, protein 5

Nut and Seed Sprinkles

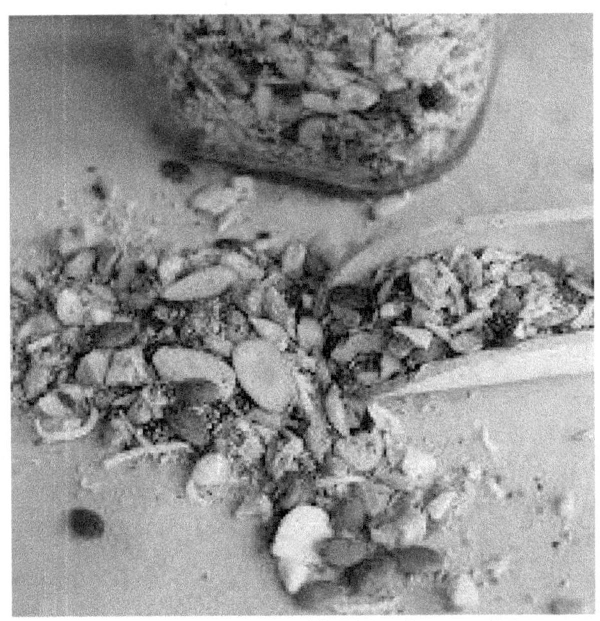

Servings: 2 cups (225 g), or 32 servings

Protein content per serving: **2 g**

Ingredients

1. 1 cup (145 g) toasted whole almonds

2. ¼ cup plus 2 tablespoons (45 g) nutritional yeast

3. ¼ cup (40 g) shelled hemp seeds

4. 1 teaspoon white miso, or scant ½ teaspoon fine sea salt, to taste

5. 1 to 2 cloves garlic, grated or pressed, to taste

6. 1½ teaspoons favorite dried herb, or a blend (dried basil, dried oregano, etc.), optional

7. ¼ teaspoon cayenne pepper, or to taste, optional

8. Direction

9. Place all the ingredients in a food processor. Pulse to combine until the almonds are coarsely ground to the consistency of panko bread crumbs.

10. Store in an airtight container in the refrigerator for up to 2 weeks.

Nutrition: calories 65, fat 1, fiber 2, carbs 6, protein 5

Almond or Cashew Biscuits

Servings: 9 biscuits

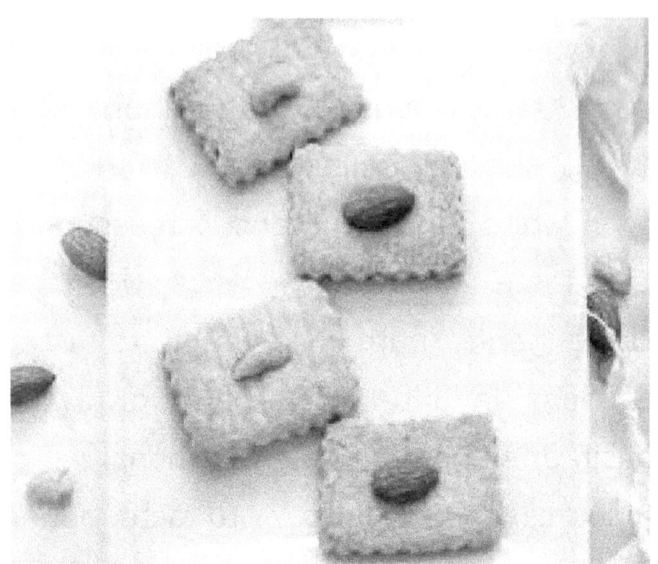

Protein content for cookie: **15 g**

Ingredients

- 1¼ cups (150 g) whole wheat pastry flour or (156 g) all-purpose flour
- ⅓ cup (47 g) toasted whole cashews or (48 g) almonds (Use unsalted.)
- ½ teaspoon fine sea salt
- 1½ teaspoons baking powder
- 1 tablespoon (42 g) semi-solid coconut oil (the texture of softened butter)

- 3 tablespoons (48 g) natural smooth cashew butter or almond butter
- ½ cup (120 g) blended soft silken tofu or unsweetened plain vegan yogurt

Direction

1. Preheat the oven to 425°F (220°C, or gas mark 7). Line a baking sheet with parch-ment paper.
2. Place the flour and nuts in a food processor. Pulse until the nuts are chopped: ¼ few larger pieces are okay. Add the salt and baking powder and pulse a couple of times.
3. Add the oil and nut butter and pulse to combine. Add the blended tofu or yogurt, and pulse until a crumbly (but not dry) dough forms. Gather the dough on a piece of parchment and pat it together to shape into a 6-inch (15 cm) square.
4. Cut into nine 2-inch (5 cm) square biscuits. Transfer the cookies to the prepared baking sheet. Bake for 12 to 14 minutes, or until golden brown at the edges cool on a wire rack and serve.

Nutrition: calories 50, fat 1, fiber 2, carbs 5, protein 5

Mushroom Cashew Mini Pies

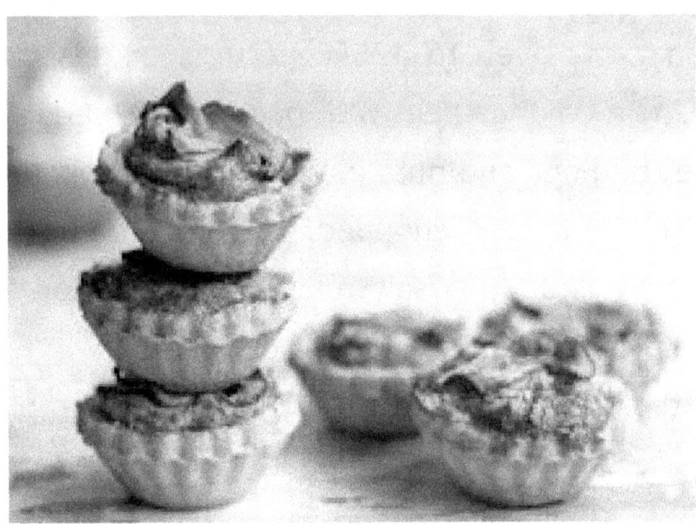

Servings: 24 mini pies

Protein content for cake: **2 g**

Ingredients

For the filling:

- 1 scant cup (210 g) Creamy Cashew Baking Spread

- 1/3 cup (80 g) minced rehydrated dried mushrooms of choice
- ¼ cup (15 g) chopped fresh parsley
- 2 tablespoons (20 g) minced red onion
- 2 tablespoons (15 g) nutritional yeast
- 2 cloves garlic, grated or pressed
- ¼ teaspoon fine sea salt
- ¼ teaspoon ground nutmeg Ground black or white pepper

For the crusts:

- Nonstick cooking spray
- 1¼ cups (150 g) whole wheat pastry flour
- ¼ cup (40 g) hemp powder
- Scant ½ teaspoon fine sea salt
- 2 tablespoons (32 g) cashew butter
- 2 tablespoons (30 ml) neutral-flavored oil
- ¼ cup plus 2 tablespoons (90 ml) cold unsweetened plain vegan milk, as needed

Direction

1. **To make the filling:** In a medium bowl, combine all the ingredients with a spoon until thoroughly mixed. Set aside while preparing the crusts.

2. **To make the crusts:** Preheat the oven to 350°F (180°C, or gas mark 4). Lightly coat a 24-cup mini muffin pan with cooking spray. Place the flour, hemp powder, and salt in a large bowl. In a small bowl, stir to combine the cashew butter and oil. Using a fork, cut the cashew butter mixture into the flour mixture. Add ¼ cup (60 ml) of the milk, stirring until crumbs form, adding an extra table-spoon (15 ml) at a time if needed. The crumbs of dough should stick together easily when pinched and be neither too dry, nor too wet.

3. Place a generous 1¼ teaspoons of crumbs in each muffin cup, pressing down to fit the bottom and sides of the bowl. Add 2 generous teaspoons of filling the per crust, smoothing out the tops.

4. Bake for 22 minutes or until the tops are firm and light golden brown. Remove from the pan, transfer to a wire rack, and serve warm or at room temperature. Leftovers can be stored in an

airtight container in the refrigerator for up to 2 days and reheated in a 325°F (170°C, or gas mark 3) oven until warm, about 15 minutes.

Nutrition: calories 150, fat 1, fiber 2, carbs 6, protein 5

Tempeh Koftas with Cashew Dip

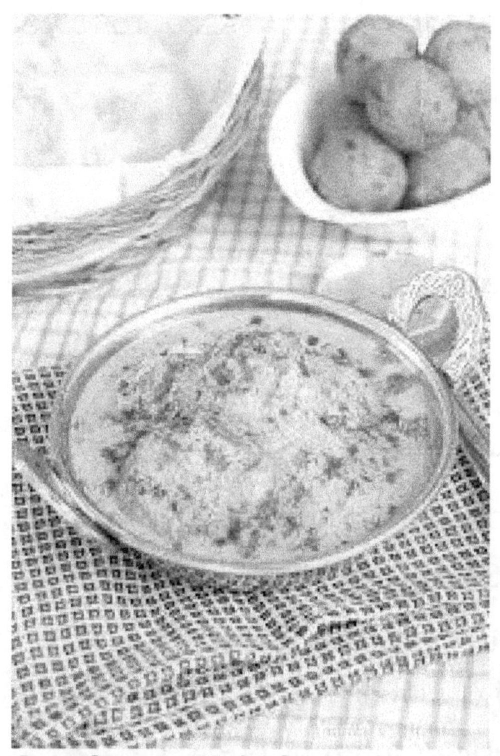

Servings: 20 koftas. plus 1 scant cup (230 g) dip

Protein content per kofta (with sauce): **6 g**

For the simple cashew dip:

- ¾ cup (180 g) cashew base
- 1½ tablespoons (6 g) packed minced fresh parsley
- 1 ¼ tablespoon (23 ml) fresh lemon juice
- 1½ tablespoons (24 g) tahini
- 1 to 2 cloves garlic, grated or pressed, to taste
- Salt and pepper

For the koftas:

- Nonstick cooking spray
- 1 cup (177 g) cannellini beans or 1 cup (171 g) black-eyed peas
- 8 ounces (227 g) tempeh
- ¾ cup (40 g) minced red onion
- ¾ cup (16 g) packed flat-leaf parsley, minced
- 2 tablespoons (30 ml) neutral-flavored oil, plus extra for brushing
- 1 tablespoon (15 g) harissa paste
- 3 large cloves garlic, grated or pressed

- 1½ teaspoons ground coriander

- 1 teaspoon ground cumin

- teaspoon fine sea salt

- ¼ teaspoon ground cinnamon

- ¼ teaspoon ground allspice

- ¼ teaspoon ground nutmeg

- 2 tablespoons (15 g) whole wheat pastry flour or (16 g) all-purpose flour

- 2 tablespoons (30 ml) fresh lemon juice, optional

- Olive oil, for brushing

Direction

1. **To make the cuttings**: 20 cups Cover a small roll of muffins with 24 cups of spray oil.

2. Grate beans or peas in a large bowl: if there are only a few beans left, that's fine. Chop the top into small pieces (do not crush). Add onions, parsley, oil. Cover the harissa paste, garlic, coriander, cumin, salt, cinnamon, spice flour, nutmeg, and flour.

3. Stir to combine. If the mixture is dry and does not come together, add the lemon juice and stir to

combine. Place a tablespoon of the round and round mixture (approximately 25 grams) on a ball and place it in a muffin pan. Repeat with the remaining bushes. Cover with a loose plastic wrap and refrigerate for 1 hour.

4. Heat the oven to 350 degrees F (180 degrees Celsius or gas mark 4).

5. Gently brush each bush with oil. Bake for 15 minutes, turn gently (fins will be brittle) and brush lightly with oil again. Bake for another 10 minutes or until golden brown.

6. Leave it on the muffin hook for 10 minutes before serving, as the soles of the foot will be brittle just outside the stove. Serve with drunken almonds. The buttercups are also delicious.

7. **For dehydration**: combine all ingredients in a food processor to combine. Occasionally, stop jamming the sides with a rubber spatula. Cover and keep for at least 1 hour in the refrigerator until ready to serve. Remnants can be stored in a refrigerated container for up to 3 days. The sink thickens after more than 24 hours after freezing.

Use it, as it spreads on bread or adds more lemon juice to taste.

Nutrition: calories 123, fat 1, fiber 8, carbs 6, protein 5

Seed and Nut Ice Cream

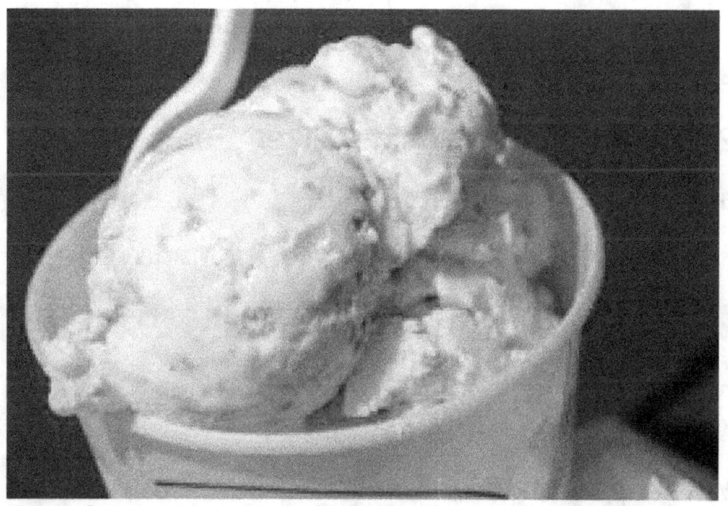

Servings: 1 quart (950 ml), or 8 servings

Protein content per serving: **9 g**

Ingredients

For the nuts:

- 1 1/3 tablespoons (30 g) pure maple syrup
- 1/3 teaspoon ground cinnamon
- ¼ teaspoon ground nutmeg
- ¼ teaspoon fine sea salt
- 1/3 cup (50 g) walnut or pecan halves
- For the ice cream:
- 1/3 cup (128 g) tahini
- ⅓ cup (128 g) natural creamy cashew butter or peanut butter
- 12 ounces (340 g) soft silken tofu, or ugly or vanilla vegan yogurt
- 1/3 cup plus 2 tablespoons (200 g) agave nectar
- ¼ cup (60 ml) full-fat coconut milk
- 1/3 teaspoon ginger powder
- 1/3 teaspoon ground cinnamon
- 1½ teaspoons pure vanilla extract

Direction

1. **To make the nuts:** Preheat the oven to 325°F (170°C, or gas mark 3).
2. In a medium bowl, mix maple syrup, cinnamon, nutmeg, and salt. Add half of the nut or walnut

and stir to foam. Place on a baking sheet with oil on a nonstick baking sheet and bake for 8 minutes. Stir for another 4 to 6 minutes to heat and dry and be careful not to dry. Before crushing, remove from oven and allow to cool completely. Set aside.

3. **To make ice cream**: Freeze your ice cream tub for at least 24 hours.

4. Put all the ingredients in the blender and mix until smooth. Try a little of the mixture to make sure it is sweet and sweet enough to your liking and, if desired, add 1 tablespoon (15 ml) at a time to the sweetener. If you make adjustments, mix again.

5. Transfer the mixture to the ice cream machine and follow the ice cream preparation Direction. Add chopped nuts during the last 5 minutes of shake. Transfer to a container and refrigerate for 2 hours. After more than a couple of hours, the ice cream does not want to be poured directly from the freezer, so let it sit for 15 minutes at room temperature.

Nutrition: calories 150, fat 1, fiber 2, carbs 5, protein 5

Chocolate Avocado Pudding

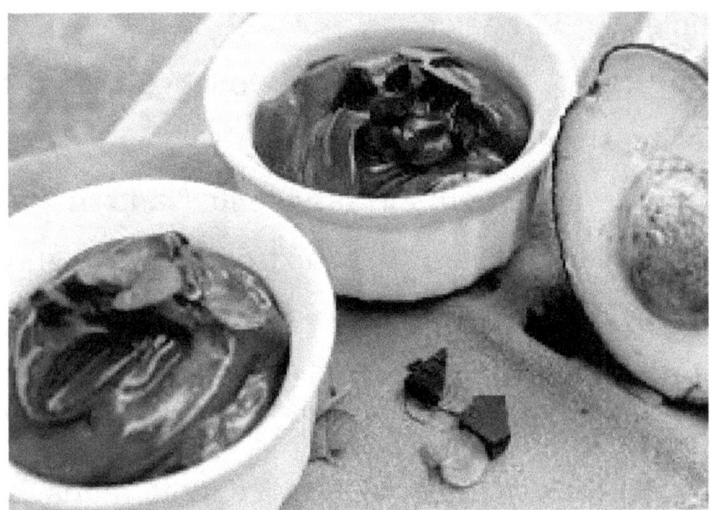

Preparation time: 30 minutes

Serves: 2

Ingredients :

- Maple syrup (quarter cup)
- Salt (pinch)
- Vanilla extract (half teaspoon)
- Almond milk (four tablespoons)

- Cocoa powder (quarter cup)
- Vegan dark chocolate chips (quarter cup)
- Ripe avocados (two medium)

Directions:

4. Heat a saucepan over medium and bring to a simmer the maple syrup and the almond milk. Take off the heat and stir in the chocolate chips to melt then set aside to cool.
5. Put everything else in a food processor then add in the milk mixture and blend until 100% smooth.
6. Spoon into individual portion containers, cover and put in the fridge until set. Enjoy!

Nutrition: calories 65, fat 1, fiber 2, carbs 4, protein 5

Decadent Chocolate Cake

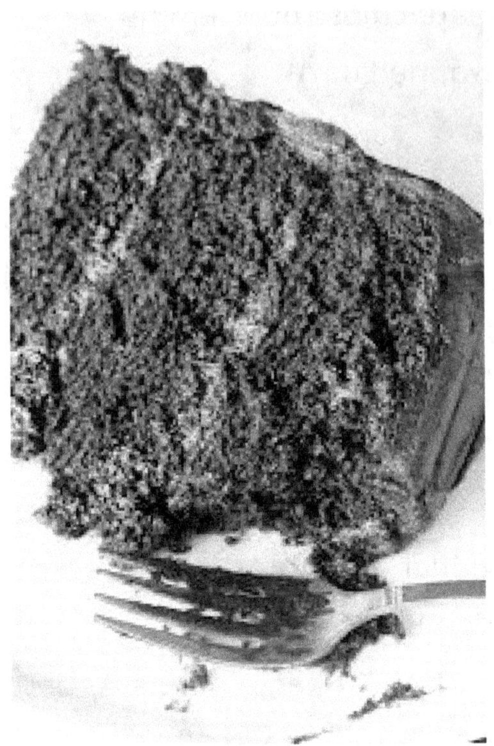

Preparation time: 30 minutes

Serves: 2

Ingredients :

- Vanilla extract (two teaspoons)
- Almond butter (two tablespoons)
- Almond milk (two and quarter cups)
- Icing sugar (two and a half cups)

- Cocoa powder (one and quarter cups)

- Dark chocolate vegan chips (quarter cups)

- Apple cider vinegar (two teaspoons)

- Vegan butter (three-quarter cup)

- Applesauce (one cup)

- Coconut oil (half cup)

- Salt (quarter cup)

- Baking powder (half teaspoon)

- Baking soda (three teaspoons)

- Raw cane sugar (one and a half cups)

- Flour (two and a half cups)

Directions:

9. Get a large bowl and sift into it the flour, baking powder, baking soda, sugar, salt and a three-quarter cup of cocoa and stir through.

10.   In a saucepan on low heat melt the coconut oil quickly then take off the heat. Put in the vinegar, one teaspoon vanilla, applesauce and two cups of the milk then mix well.

11.   Put everything together and mix with an electric beater until it's really smooth.

12.   Pour into two 8-inch cake pans lined with baking paper and bake for forty-five minutes at 350F. Check by inserting a knife to the center at an angle, if the knife is clean when you remove it, then it is cooked through. Leave to cool.

13.   In a clean saucepan, melt together the vegan butter and chocolate chips on low heat while stirring.

14.   In a bowl, sift in the rest of the cocoa powder with the icing sugar, one teaspoon vanilla, almond butter and the rest of the almond milk. Pour in the chocolate butter and mix with an electric beater until thick and creamy.

15.   Slice the very top off of one cake to make it flat and spoon some frosting on top. Spread it around before adding the second cake. Ice the entire double-stacked cake with the rest of the icing, starting with the top and then moving the icing down around the edges.

16.   Sprinkle the top with whatever you like! Chocolate shavings or shredded coconut, chopped nuts or berries. Enjoy!

Nutrition: calories 54, fat 1, fiber 2, carbs 6, protein 5

Conclusion

In this cookbook, you have been provided with the crucial information you need to know about the vegan lifestyle, how to plan out balanced meals with all the nutrients your body requires, the most helpful and healthy Ingredients to include in your daily life, tips, and tricks to make the lifestyle simple to follow and recipes!

Not only have you gained over recipes to help you enjoy the plant-based lifestyle to the fullest, you have also gained tips and tricks to make the changes easier, a list of important Ingredients you can include in your daily life, information on how to create balanced meals without animal-based products, and the basics about the vegan lifestyle including reasons why to go vegan. Whether you are going vegan to improve your health, decrease animal cruelty, do your part to lessen climate change or all the above, you will find that with these recipes, you can attain your goal.

Making a lifestyle change can appear daunting. After all, we already have to deal with enough stress in our daily lives, so changing our regular routine can seem overwhelming. However, with an understanding of the vegan lifestyle, meal planning, and this collection of simple and delicious recipes, you will be able to easily make a change for the better and follow the vegan lifestyle with ease. You don't have to love, or even be good at, cooking to be good at meal prepping. You'll definitely find that your knife skills will improve as you cut, chop, and prepare meals each week, but don't be intimidated if you're not spending a lot of time in your kitchen. Plenty of vegans survive on takeout from restaurants and grocery store packages, but if you really want to take control of your diet, meal prep is the way to go.

If you are trying to change your lifestyle, it calls for immense commitment and hard work. It is quite easy to fall for loopholes and give up early or even halfway through because you cannot find the energy and motivation to handle the changes.

Set yourself easy to achieve targets initially. Setting unachievable targets can put you off as you see yourself as a failure. Take a little at a time and be motivated by your small achievements. Slowly, you will see setting higher targets and achieve them too.

Becoming a vegan may not be an easy fear, particularly if you are a meat-lover.

But if you will consider all the benefits that it can bring to your health, and at the same time, how this lifestyle helps animals, it would be much easier to set your mind to make the transition.

Remember, you do not have to do it drastically. You can start gradually, and then by the time you have made the switch; you will start to experience all the wonderful benefits that veganism can bring to your life. Now that you have a better idea of how you'll be meal prepping each week, your journey as a vegan can be a much less complicated.